What Sam's Colleagues, Friends and Family are Saying About *I Love What I Do!*

Sam—you've done it! I've long admired you—your music, drumming and singing. But more: not just your life in life, but your life as music—joyous and beautiful. Your wonderful style of living.

And now you've encapsulated its essence in this very inspiring and necessary book. I heartily recommend it to all who, regardless of age and musical experience, really want to LIVE.

To this end, I've recommended to many depressives that they should call your phone number—just to listen to your recorded message. Your voice, and of course, your music, is so uplifting, so therapeutic.

And so too is your life-enhancing book.

Dr. John Diamond, M.D.
The Way of the Pulse: Drumming With Spirit

Sam Ulano is a man dedicated to his art and sharing his knowledge. This book is a testament to that fact.

Mike Farriss
Director of Artistic Relations, Pearl Corporation

Having known Sam Ulano for over 40 years, I have admired him as much for his independent spirit and positive philosophy as his many musical accomplishments. Many younger (and older) people could well benefit from reading this inspiring book—congratulations, Sam...Glad we're friends.

Ed Shaughnessy
Six-time winner "Best Big Band Drummer",
Modern Drummer Poll
29 years playing on "The Johnny Carson Show"

Sam Ulano has taught me about life in general as well as teaching me about playing [the drums], teaching [them] and the music business [as a whole]. Thanks Sam!

> Tony Monforte, Tony Monforte Drum School
> Drummer for Pat "the Cat" Band

Rarely have I met a drummer who is as straight-forward and dedicated to the art of drum kit instruction as Sam.

Sam's philosophy and instruction technique are core basics, and emphasize what most drummers overlook as the essential tools to excelling in the drum kit playing area.

> Andy Zildjian, Sabian Cymbal Makers

As far as drum playing, drum instruction and drum writing goes, there is no one on the scene that can match Sam's accomplishments.

My brother Sam is the finest drum instructor, the finest drummer, and the most prolific writer of drum books of the century. He has many CD's and Video recordings available.

Having said all that, I can only say that the drum world will agree with all that I have written about Sam.

I, too, am a musician, having run an Accordion School and having played for the past fifty years. I feel completely at ease when I say Sam is one of the greatest in his field.

I have had occasion to attend various affairs where orchestras have performed, from Boston to Miami. Every drummer in every band I spoke with either knows Sam personally, having studied with him, or are using his written material for their teaching purposes. Sam is the best, no doubt about it.

God bless you, Sam, and keep it up until you are 100.

> Ben Olanoff, (Sam's brother)

Renowned drum educator and innovator, Sam Ulano, shares his over 80 years of life and music business experience, told from the perspective of a no-frills loving father.

> Phil Bloom
> Fellow Drum Educator and Performer

Truly inspiring. After more than 60 years as an educator of generations of musicians, Sam Ulano gives us a glimpse of some of his secrets for living a rich, healthy and satisfying life.

Stephen Korbel
Student, Musician and Corporate Executive

Sam is truly the happiest person I have ever met, and I have known him for 47 years.

Mark Ulano, (Sam's son)

During the years I've worked with Sam Ulano, he has become my friend and, as a bonus, the fine musician I often play with. This order has reversed over the years. When I first worked with Sam, we were the rhythm section. As we continued to work together, he became a friend whom I have come to admire and then an extraordinary musician whom I have come to respect. He lives his philosophy, and gladly shares it with his students, fellow band members, casual visitors to the venues where he works, and anyone who is lucky enough to be around him for any length of time.

Leonard Gaskin, Bassist

Mr. Ulano's book is a delight, packed with practical wisdom delivered in an upbeat manner. He is a "drummer's drummer" with an appealing, positive philosophy for each "swinging" day.

Al Warner, Ph.D.
Musician & Counselor

Sam Ulano's philosophy of life can be summed up in a drumshell...Life is what happens while you are playing other gigs...Enjoy the moment...Become the moment...Be in the moment...Keep swingin' Sam!

Russ Moy
Drummer, Educator and Clinician

Sam Ulano is a unique individual who abides by his own laws of decency, self-education, strict body discipline and moral ethics. This has resulted in a miraculous human being with a sense of humor who is a role model for young and old alike.

He has raised his own bar many times and has exceeded his high standards with his many accomplishments—musician, teacher, author, philosopher and—more to come, I am sure.

I am pleased to be known as "Sam Ulano's oldest living student"—having known this National Treasure for over 50 years!

Arthur "Artie" Scher

Sam Ulano is a consummate professional, both on and off the bandstand. He approaches everything with joy, and his love of people, of life, of music, of the audience, and of his fellow musicians has made him a role model for myself and nearly everyone who knows him.

Ed Polcer

If you ever have the pleasure of meeting Sam Ulano, you will know that his philosophy works. He is one of the most vital, productive and happy people I've ever known. If the world was full of people living Sam's philosophy of life, it would be a much more joyous place!!

Michael Greenberg, CSW, ACSW

Sam Ulano's book *I Love What I Do! A Drummers Philosophy of Life at 80* is a great book for everyone. His philosophies are timeless and cross all boundaries of age and culture. He tells it like it is in plain English, which makes it easy for everyone to read and comprehend. The format that he uses is ingenious. You can read what you choose and refer back effortlessly as needed. I highly recommend Sam's book!!

Stephen Stone

Since I have been studying drums under Sam Ulano, he has opened many doors to my potential as a drummer, teacher, and businessman. His teaching methods get results and they remain fresh after even 60 years of drum instruction. The philosophy that he presents in this book will prove to be practical and inspirational.

Raymond Levitt,
Drummer, Percussionist, & Educator

The Great French Philosopher Descartes said, "I think therefore I am." I have known Sam Ulano for over forty years and studied with him at different times. In his book Sam's philosophy comes through loud and clear, "I <u>think</u> and <u>swing</u> therefore I am." It is well known that Sam is one of the best readers in the business, and that he has great chops. In this book he tells us how he got there, and remains there at age eighty.

David A. Shapiro, M.D.
Associate Professor of Psychiatry

The name Sam Ulano has resounded for generations in the music world—but his "words of wisdom," so wonderfully articulated in his *Philosophy of Life,* can be appreciated universally.

In Sam's inimitable style, he enlightens or reminds us—on every page—of the common sense approach to work and life. You can read it over and over and it still feels fresh. A treasure for everyone!

Allan S. Colin, President
Charles Colin Publications

As a psychiatrist, I believe your book *I Love What I Do!* can be used as a primer for living one's life. It is written with grace and humor. As a <u>tribal elder,</u> your thoughts are profound, meaningful, useful and presented in an eye-twinkling humorous style that is unique to Sam Ulano.

It's uplifting to see the logic of living life written by one who has lived it so well. You remain my personal drumchiatrist. Thanks for sharing your wisdom over the past years.

Eugene M. Kornhaber, P.C.

Sam Ulano knows the power of positive music. He will play your 100th birthday.

Phil Schapp, WKCR-FM Radio Station

Sam's book is a wonderful expression of the importance of believing in your self.

Thomas Olin, Cats—Titanic
Illinois Jacquet's Big Band

Sam's "Philosophy of Life" book gives not only the drummer, but all who read its pages a wholesome and positive direction. It's a complete guide for young and old in how to make it all happen. All the best.

Bill Rotella, Rotella Drum Studio

Sam's book is great—simple, practical and profound wisdom that we can all live by!

Like Sam's book, studying drums with him provides not only a wealth of information dealing with drums but a very personal approach that has helped me tremendously. Thanks Sam!

James Guarnieri, Performing Artist
Music Educator/Band Director

Sam Ulano's contribution and devotion to the World of Drumming are unprecedented. As a teacher and author, his achievements are many. His "No Frills" approach to teaching and writing effectively deals with the real issues that face professional drummers. *I Love What I Do!* is a book comprised of 80 years of wisdom rolled into one journal, which you will not find in any other text to date on the subject of Drumming. This book is a must read for all who are seeking a proven method for success as a drummer. I am very lucky to know and have studied with Sam Ulano. The Drumming World is extremely lucky to have a Sam Ulano.

Gene Jackson
Herbie Hancock's Band

Aside from being a good guy, Sam was (and is) a joy to work with. A swinging drummer with great taste, not to mention marvelous technique and an encyclopedic knowledge of any and all rhythms.

As you will read in this book, Sam personifies qualities which we all admire. He wants us all to try to be professional in every way as he is—including the "little things" like being on time, looking presentable, cooperating, learning the tunes, etc. Working with Sam has helped me tremendously!

Dick Brady "Trombonist Supreme" (according to Sam)
Numerous bands, including Glen Miller's and Kay Kyser's

In this personal, life-affirming monograph, Mr. Ulano shares with his readers the commonsense principles and simple home truths that have guided him through nearly eight decades of achievement and distinction as a performer, teacher, writer and record producer. Open the book anywhere—it doesn't matter. Every page is an ode "l'chayim."

Bruce Macomber
Editor/Writer

Your book is filled with many ideas that people can follow to enrich their lives. The main theme that shines through is your steady dedication toward improving yourself in your field. Having dedication to a cause helps one to manage throughout the years.

Wishing you all the best and success with the book.

Sol (Sam's brother, also 80)

I will always be grateful to Sam Ulano for teaching me to believe in myself, and to understand the importance of working hard for what we love, and that with perseverance and focus we can achieve just about anything we put our minds to. Thank-you Sam!

Richie Rodriguez
Drum Educator, Performer, Author

Many people regard Sam Ulano as a guru of education, a "<u>drumcologist</u>"! Sam personifies the true meaning of "<u>living legend</u>" through his pursuit in mastering the many intense aspects of life. Control and discipline have driven Sam to always be a step ahead of the rest.

Throughout my 33 years of knowing Sam, he's never ceased to amaze me through his positive and motivating attitude towards life. His teachings and concepts are the most useful and practical of all the methods I've experienced. At the age of 80, Sam's philosophy is truly <u>timeless</u>, <u>honest</u> and <u>witty</u>! Bravo—Sam!!

John Sarracco

Some excellent ideas for a happy professional, personal…successful life are contained in this book.

Ida, "Sam's Sister, age 95"

Although Sam Ulano's opinions are radical and unique, he can back them up with the most prized of all accomplishments in the music business, longevity. His 68 years of drumming has included educating some of the finest drummers, performances in the top NYC jazz clubs, the NYC school system, on many television shows and recordings, and everything in between. His books share the insight that can only be gained by a lifetime of making music. His teachings will open your ears to a creative new outlook on drumming, while focusing on versatility, musicality, and the beauty of the drum set. The drum and music industries owe a great deal of thanks to Mr. Rhythm, Sam Ulano.

Mark Griffith, Recording Artist, Drum Historian
Featured Writer for Stick It, Modern Drummer, and Batteur

There is a teacher for everyone—for the *serious* student there is only Sam Ulano. My love to you Sam.

Azande Cummins, Drummer and Drum Educator

Another great philosopher once said that the true function of education is to provide a "toolbox of ideas" that you can use to live your life. Sam Ulano's Philosophy of Life is exactly that: it is the distillation of an 80-year search for a system that really works. This wonderful book contains suggestions and guidance on the kinds of issues that face each of us every day, but which nobody ever really talks about. This is what they should really teach in schools.

> Paul Cavaciuti, Music for Health Practitioner
> Drummer, Former Head of PIT, London

What can I say about Sam? He always speaks his mind and never wastes time. He taught me to be me, which is not always easy. He helped me to sing with bands. I think he's great—love you Sam.

> Corky "D" Romash, Band Vocalist

Just finished reading a draft of your latest book, and it looks like a real winner. You are truly a multi-talented individual as well as a living jazz legend. I wish you all the best. Keep on swingin'…

> Vin Piraino

Congratulations on your upcoming book publication. It is the culmination of all your professional life, and another tribute to your dedication to it. From your boyhood through the years of your military service in the 398th Infantry—years of entertaining, near and far, always teaching, writing and believing in yourself and your students—the Ulano's have taken pride in your accomplishments. We send our love and best wishes— may you enjoy success and good health.

> Sarah (Sam's Sister) and Family

I *Love* What I Do!

A Drummer's Philosophy of Life at Eighty

Sam Ulano

ENHANCEMENT BOOKS
Bloomingdale, Illinois

I Love What I Do! A Drummer's Philosophy of Life at Eighty
Copyright 2001 by Sam Ulano

Published by: Enhancement Books
                P.O. Box 544
                Bloomingdale, IL 60108
                Website: www.vitalhealth.net
                E-mail: vitalhealth@compuserve.com

Printed in the United States of America

ISBN 1-890995-35-5

Table of Contents

Sam Ulano's Approach
to Getting Better and Reaching Goals

At the age of 80, I've finally decided to put on paper my concepts for living. This is something I've always wanted to do. Recently it came to me how I would do this: I would simply start writing and hope that, in the end, some of the knowledge I've gained in eight decades is of some value to you reading it.

All my life I've been a drummer, both student and educator. I somehow always had the ability to teach others. I also had the talent to demonstrate and explain to my students why and how the study material I developed could benefit them. This must have worked because so many people I taught are still playing and are in the music profession, where drum study was essential to them.

The following ideas are what I have found to have worked for me. I like to think of them as my ideas for living. I pass them on to you so you might make use of these concepts and have the use of my past experience. This doesn't mean that they will work for you. But they might provide some direction that can help you. Although most of these concepts have been written about by others, maybe I can give you another slant on things.

With the possible exception of the first chapter on developing a system, this book doesn't have to be read straight-through. Instead, see which topics are relevant to you and check out my experience with them. You never know when some outside mind may give you a new approach to how you can better yourself. Above all, keep in mind that this is a book about music—about life—as I see it from eight decades.

Study these ideas for living and try to apply them. If they work for you, then I'm glad to have helped. If they don't, then keep searching and looking for what works for you. The key is to never stop learning!

Yours for a better life and more fun in living your life, I remain,

Sam Ulano, *the Drumchiatrist*

Developing a System

It took me many years to come to the conclusion that I had to develop a system for my life. I was living a system, of course, but in the early stages of my life, I didn't know it. I think many of us don't realize that we are living some sort of system. We can have a good system or a bad system, or rather, one that helps us meet our goals or one that doesn't. How do we know if our plan for life is good or bad? The results we get will tell us. Just remember it takes time to develop a feel for what works and what doesn't.

Routine plays a big role in any system. I have a routine of when I sleep and when I wake up. When I go to work. Who studies with me. The time the student has to show up. What level the student is at. All these facts come into play when I teach. I've been teaching for so many years that it comes naturally to me, and I just know what, where and with whom I am involved.

As with any routine, there must be a starting point to your daily life. I'm a big believer in this idea. You just can't get up in the morning (or whenever you wake up) and think the day starts without a definite plan. If this sounds rigid to you, then so be it. However, I really feel we must be organized. You can't go about your day helter-skelter.

One of the reasons big business, supermarkets, the stock market, the police department, the army, navy and successful people make it is that they have a plan—a system. Whether the method they use is working or not, at least they work with a definite plan. I will use these two words a lot: system and plan. For the most part, they are one and the same.

As for me, 80 years have taught me that I need a system to cover three very important areas of my life:

- my health
- my education
- my finances

Think about these. They may not be important to you now, but they should be. For without good health, we are in trouble. We will find it difficult to get up day after day and do what our talents want us to do. Without education, or learning, we cannot develop our abilities to communicate, to keep our minds sharp, or to grow in our chosen field of endeavor. As for finances, I don't need to tell you that you can't ride the bus for free. Not even at 80!

Thus, these are the three parts of my life to which I steadfastly apply a plan. As you continue reading, you'll notice that most of my concepts for success revolve around these three areas. Of course, when I was a young man, I didn't understand any of these areas. But we all grow up and eventually learn about them. As we mature, we realize that health, education, and finances are the building blocks for everything else.

YOU ONLY GET ONE LIFE

Remember that you have one set of eyes. You have one set of ears. You have only one body that was given to you and you must train it and take care of it. It's the only one you have or are going to get. When I was 22, I was drafted into the army. This was during World War II and I learned a great deal about my physical body. Then, a funny thing happened. I was discharged and I forgot all I had learned. After getting married, I fell completely out of shape, and by the time I was 40, I had ballooned to 320 pounds! I hadn't realized that I wasn't taking care of the one body that I had.

Fortunately, a student of mine introduced me to a gym on the corner of the block where I had my drum studio. This chap took me to Sigmond Klien's gym, and with the help of Sigmond Klien himself, I was taught how to train with weights. Soon I lost 130 pounds. I've stayed with that body conditioning routine ever since. Today, I weigh 177 pounds and train with light weights every day. I never miss a day. I've written a chapter about how and why I use the weights in my body development program. This may give you some important ideas to help you.

Remember I speak of this at the age of 80. BUT THAT DOESN'T MEAN I'M FINISHED LEARNING. I'm now developing my ideas on how I'll stay in shape to reach a healthy 90 years. Not only to keep my body healthy, but my mind as well. One thing is sure: The system I have works and I am confident it can work for anyone who wants to be healthy and happy with their lives.

So I have a system for keeping my body well. One way to do this is to remember the adage, you are what you eat. I couldn't agree more with the person who discovered this connection between the food we eat and the person we are. When I say stay in good health, I mean above all to watch your food intake. If you can't come up with a good system for eating, see a food nutritionist; it's money well spent. But once you walk out the door, even a food nutritionist can't help you exert control over your food choices. Only you can do that.

As for me, I have—you guessed it—a system. You'll see tidbits of this system expressed throughout this book. In short, I don't eat much dairy food. I don't eat meals after seven o'clock at night. I try very hard not to eat anything before I go to bed. I eat very little fried foods. I try not to eat too much meat. I do eat fish, lobster, pasta, cake, and even use a little butter on my bread. I drink very little milk and soda. I don't smoke and I very rarely drink alcohol. Basically, I eat all types of food, because I enjoy them. But here's the catch: I eat them in MODERATION. The main ingredient in my diet is that I eat WITH CONTROL. I'm not going to lie to you and say it's easy, but it can be done! Because of this key, I can honestly say that I have never felt better in my life.

Now let me give you a little insight into my health. I am a diabetic, type 2. This means I take a tablet every day called Glipazide. I understand this controls my blood sugar. Keeping a healthy weight is so very important to diabetics. I also had skin melanoma 15 years ago. I was operated on at the VA Hospital here in New York shortly after it was diagnosed and the doctors have watched me like a hawk since then. I go in for regular check-ups, and so far I am cancer-free.

So at this point in my life, I have my weight under control, my diabetes under control, and my skin cancer too. It feels great to be on top of these physical problems. I listen to my doctors. They are the ones who know how to handle these problems, so I listen. As a student of my instrument, I've always been a good listener.

KNOW WHAT'S IMPORTANT AND ADAPT

Another part of my system for life is my practice time and how I stay on top of my professional life. I must practice every day. It's a must in my life. I get two, three or as many hours of practice time in as possible. I never miss a day. I know how to practice, why I practice, and what to practice.

My drumming career is important. The main thrust of my percussion practice is spent developing my music reading. I spend many hours on my reading skills. Reading is so important. This is of utmost importance in developing my drum abilities. Without reading a person will become a dumb drummer. We learn to read and write because this is how we can communicate with each other. If you can't read, you can't play with a big band. You can't play the classics. You can't teach others about so many parts of music.

Also important in my system is what I do with my free time. I know that there are 24 hours in each day. We must sleep some of the time. We must eat, take care of our personal habits. We must have a certain amount of time to socialize with our friends and spend time with our families. We need time to study and time to work so we can earn a living to pay our bills.

In my system I have time for everything I need and wish to do. I somehow divide my 24 hours so I can cover all the bases in my life. My system is very organized—for me. This doesn't mean it is how you will live your life. I develop what works for Sam Ulano. I live with myself and know who I am and what works for me. Everything in my life must be organized. EVERYTHING I WORK AT SHOULD WORK.

While my system for each day is pretty much the same, I am flexible to be able to change with what happens. Or as they say, I go with the flow. For instance, many times I get a gig at the last minute. These are the things that go with the territory. We must change with the changes.

Create a system. Roll with the punches. Change what needs to be changed. You operate under a system even now, whether you know it or not. Why not make it work for you? Use it to help you do all the things you want to do.

Study Only With People Who Know How to Teach

To become someone who really knows their craft you must search for an educator who knows what to teach and offers a professional level of instruction. That person should be able to give you a definite program of study.

Somebody once said, "Amateurs teach amateurs; professionals teach professionals." I agree with this. I have always studied with people who were active in the business of music. An educator that has information who could steer the student in the proper direction. A no-nonsense educator who has lived the life of a working musician. To me, these are the only people who know and can direct the pupil in the true sense of the word, as a person who knows what really works.

When I was looking for an instructor, I would ask a teacher to play for me. One educator asked me why I wanted to hear him play. My reply was THAT I WANTED TO HEAR WHAT I WOULD SOUND LIKE AFTER STUDYING WITH HIM. If he didn't play for me, I would turn around and leave and seek out someone who would play for me and explain what we would work on. This information gave me some definite direction as to where this teacher was coming from.

A word here on "music teachers." Because an instructor is at the high school or college level of teaching music doesn't mean this person is a good instructor. Most school teachers involved with music can't play their instrument. They're in school almost ten hours a day and have no time to practice. After years in the school system, if these teachers were ever any good, their talents have eroded from lack of practice and honing their skills.

The true professional in the world of music says beware of a person who is in the school system NO MATTER WHAT LEVEL OF EDUCATION. These people have stopped studying their instrument and their abilities have eventually deteriorated. It's true.

Stay on Top of Your Practice

This is important if you are ever to gain control of your abilities. Many of us make excuses for why we can't find the time to practice. See if any of these sound familiar:

> I had to go back to school...My grandmother took very sick...I had to work past my regular hours because there were things that had to be done...One of the other workers didn't show...I was on vacation...My wife wanted to see a movie...My kids had some problems...The car had to get fixed.

On and on the excuses go. I know we all have problems, but we should look at our daily lives and see where we can fit in our serious practice time.

I look at each day and set my goals as to how much practice I can get in. I TRY MY BEST TO NEVER LET OUTSIDE THINGS DISRUPT MY DAILY LIFE, so that I stick to my routine of organized practice time. At 80 years old I maintain a steady diet of training. I believe that if I stay on top of my practice time I will be in the best playing ability. I don't want to allow myself to lose my abilities after 68 years of hard study. Besides, the payoff—sounding the way I want to sound—is worth it.

I say to all my students that I can only take care of my talent. And each of you can only take care of your own. To do so, each of us must develop our own systems of training. And stay on top of it.

Don't Overeat

Eating is one of the most important parts of our lives. Controlling what we take into our bodies is incredibly important. I speak from past experience. As I wrote in the first chapter, I was as heavy as 320 pounds when I reached 40 years old. I wasn't aware of how out of condition I'd become. Thankfully, I caught myself before it was too late, back in 1960, and I did something about it. I came up with a method of eating and exercising my body. Being out of shape is very dangerous, and I feel I was smart about making a change. Forty years later, I've stayed on top of my physical makeup.

I do not ever want to be 320 pounds or even close to that awful condition I was in. It was a terrible state of my life and I'm glad I did something about it. It might not have felt great while developing the discipline to change, but it feels great now. At 80 years old, I know I did the right thing.

As I wrote elsewhere, MODERATION IN EVERYTHING I DO is the key to my success. That holds especially true for eating, because eating for most of us is a pleasurable experience. We might feel like we don't know when to stop. Believe me, we know. Approach your meals with the idea of moderation in mind, every day, and it will be easier to listen to your body. You'll feel better in the short-term because you'll have extra energy from not having to digest all that food, and you'll feel good in the long-run because you'll still have your body with which to do things.

Don't Believe Those
Who Aren't Tops in Their Fields

In my opinion, those who are not among the best in their fields are not good role models for those of us who wish to learn and develop our talents. I am skeptical of people who tell others how to be top quality talents in their chosen work when they haven't experienced the type of success they are telling us about.

I do not cloud my methods of instruction with so much nonsense and hide behind the fact I have a reputation in my musical life. As I've evolved as a teacher, I have done away with traditional drum studies, even though my fellow drum instructors still hold onto much of the early drum instruction from many years gone by. Much of the traditional basic drum study has nothing to do with really playing the drums in these times.

Someone once said a photo is sometimes better than a thousand words. I feel the same about DEMONSTRATING HOW SOMETHING SHOULD BE DONE. That demonstration can many times clear up drum studies for my students. Now, of course, not all instructors can demonstrate the final results of a page of music. But a good teacher can explain in words why certain things are done and how to do them.

I feel I have the ability to explain and perform what I am teaching. My students get a better understanding of how to play a particular study book. In fact, when I write a book about certain drum ideas, I always make sure I give a clear and definite word picture of what the book is about. I can explain why I wrote the book and where and when the material in the study work is to be used, either in teaching or live performances.

Real life to me is living my life and being able to tell someone what I experienced in my musical career and why I teach the way I do.

Don't Eat Before Going to Bed

I found a very important part of my life was keeping my weight down. Being a DIABETIC, this is one of the keys to living better and longer. Ask any nutritionist and they will tell you that not eating close to bedtime is a very important part of feeling good and preventing yourself from being overweight.

One of the methods I use is NOT EATING BEFORE I GO TO BED. Once I had this under control, I found I felt a lot like getting up in the morning and getting my work done. In addition, I don't feel bloated, like I want to go to the bathroom and sit on the pot. I stop eating at about seven or eight o'clock in the evening. Many times I cut my food intake at about six. It took me some time to get used to this, but I eventually mastered it.

I also don't eat before I go out to perform with my band. Not eating before playing my instrument means that I can use my stomach muscles for playing the drums. If I feel I must eat before playing a gig, it will be something very light: a salad or soup and a cup of coffee. I don't eat much bread and butter. As a result, I feel great and have control of my body and can play my instrument.

Many times I watch the fellows in my band overeat and I don't think they are relaxed and don't feel they have the complete mastery over their abilities. This is just my opinion. I do not claim this is the same for everyone. I just state this for Sam Ulano—it works for me. I've watched fellow musicians put a steak away. Or a hamburger with a big order of french fries, covered with salt, pepper, ketchup and mustard, and a large salad. I know I can't do that and I don't do that.

You'll Pay the Price
Even If You Don't Pay the Price

Someone once asked me what I meant by that statement. I mean that if you don't take care, you'll not be well-trained and will pay the price by not being prepared in your life for whatever may come along. Both the good things and the not-so-good things.

If you wish to get better, you have to invest in yourself. LITERALLY, YOU HAVE TO PAY THE PRICE. This means paying for lessons, books, equipment, proper clothes—the tools of your trade, no matter what they may be. If you don't get what you need ahead of time, you'll pay the price down the road. Like the Boy Scouts, we must always be ready. Be prepared. This is very important.

As a musician, I need a tuxedo, two black suits, shirts, ties, bowties. As a drummer, I need a good set of drums. These things are musts. In addition, I need business cards, professional photos, a press kit, and maybe some microphones, a sound system and other items that I may be called upon to bring to a job.

However, YOU ALSO HAVE TO PAY THE PRICE FIGURATIVELY.

My mother always used to say if you stop being a student, you are finished as a true professional. By this she meant one must always practice and study and keep on top of their craft. You can never let your talents flounder and allow yourself not to be on top of your talents. You must always be learning.

Take lessons all the time, get new books, and develop your abilities. We don't know what tomorrow will bring and just when opportunities may come. If you are not ready, you'll pay the price in the form of lost opportunities. Even then, if you decide to put the work in, there will be a price to pay—in the form of the study and preparedness you neglected.

I hope I cleared that up!

Read Lots of Books

One important thing about all forms of study is there's a great deal of literature on all topics and all levels of interest. What I did (and still do) is put aside some of the money I make from various gigs, even if it is only a dollar, and I save up until I have enough to buy books. In my case, I buy music books. But anyone can and should find books on their particular areas of interest. Books and knowledge are the key for all of us to progress toward our goals.

After all, most knowledge is in books: They cover ideas we need to know. Studying these concepts day in and day out adds up to a wealth of knowledge. Try, just for a day, measuring your "wealth" in terms of knowledge rather than dollars. Then try it again tomorrow. And the day after that. Pretty soon you might feel like you don't know all the answers. That should get you thinking differently!

Reading for me has had another benefit: I have done a great deal of writing about my instrument. I try to cover areas that others haven't developed. I write about both musical concepts and practical ideas that I feel are important. Yet, it's funny that with all my writing and what everyone else has written about the study of drums, THERE'S STILL SO MUCH MATERIAL THAT HAS NOT BEEN WRITTEN ABOUT.

In every field of endeavor there are people writing and adding to what has been done over the years. This makes sense to me. When I came along at the age of 13, there was very little study material for drums. A few classical books. Very little about playing on the drum set as we know it today. I'm certain this exists in all areas—technology, finance, the arts. But all over the world people are thinking, writing and helping all of us to learn.

In addition, nowadays there's the Internet, computers, videos, CDs, DVDs and all kinds of forms of information. But how do we think these things came about? From LEARNING AS MUCH AS WE CAN ON A SUBJECT and then applying what we've learned and adding to it. Just think of what lies on the horizon!

You'll hear me say this throughout this book whenever education comes up, but if doctors operated on us in 2000 the way they did in 1940, many of us would be dead. So books and knowledge are the keys for all of us to progress toward our goals.

Take an Interest in Your Own Life

It's very interesting. I never thought that I would be writing my ideas about how I think and what I feel would make us better. When I was very young going to public school, I wasn't a very good student. In fact, I was terrible. Never studied and never read a book. I was poor in math and very poor in English. Didn't study history, geography or any subject. Of course, in later years when I wanted to become a drummer and be in the percussion field, I suffered because I didn't know anything.

As I said earlier, I paid the price later on for not paying the price. I was fortunate, though, because people like Mr. Aubry Brooks and some of my school music educators saw that I had a special talent for music. THEY DIRECTED ME INTO THINKING AND LEARNING WHAT I HAD TO KNOW TO DEVELOP AS A PROFESSIONAL MUSICIAN.

Being a serious student and having the ability to think and want to get better, I learned how to listen to people. In my army days in the band, I was most fortunate to meet Phil Bodner, who was one of the few members of the band who knew the world of music. He helped me so much in my younger days as a growing musician.

Then when I went to the Manhattan School of Music I studied with the great Dr. Alfred Friezie as one of his timpani students. He helped me understand the timpani. How to practice, what to practice, and how to use this instrument in my career. It was a very important part of my life.

As I grew older, I realized I was fortunate to come from a large family. I'm a twin. And my mother had another set of twins ahead of my twin brother and me. My oldest brother Joseph Ulano invented the silk screen process. He was a genius. My sisters were very encouraging to me by always telling me to improve my English and math skills and to always study.

In my early days as a young and growing person, my sisters and older brothers instilled great values in me. Not to waste my time. To always learn whatever I needed to learn. To control my dollars and many other valuable concepts of life.

At first I didn't understand these ideas, but like many of us, as the mind develops, we eventually start to understand and know where we are coming from. We learn how to develop our lives in more than just one area. To me, this all became clear, and I really found what I wanted out of my life. At the age of 80, this all makes sense to me. I was better off because of all of this help I received along the way. And yet all of this interest in me wouldn't have meant a thing *if I didn't show an interest in myself.*

Make Decisions

I'm a big believer that we must learn to make definite decisions. You can't work a system without being certain what you plan to do and what you need to do. You can't decide to go left and then decide to go right. This can be very dangerous. Go with your gut feelings and don't be wishy-washy about what you are going to do.

Being indecisive can give other people the feeling you don't know what you want to get done in your life. When I make a decision, I carry it out to the fullest. I can't stand not being final in what I wish to do. Whether it's in my time to practice my instrument or paying my bills, I can't have all these loose ends hanging around. When I tell myself to do something, I do it and get it out of my way. Then I do the next thing that I feel is important.

Definite direction can be so rewarding and make me feel good about myself. Try it and see how you feel. GET IT DONE AND OUT OF THE WAY; THE SOONER, THE BETTER.

In my early days I never had control over my decisions. However, once I learned how to do this I was so happy and had lots of time for more important things.

Sometimes the things we make decisions about are very minor things that must be done. But we sometimes procrastinate and do not take care of these little items we need to take care of. We just hang onto them. All of a sudden we find the little things become mountainous and get out of control. Don't let this happen to you. Stay on top of your decisions. MAKE THEM AND TAKE CARE OF THEM. It's very important to making your life interesting and exciting.

Be Yourself

I think it is important that we be ourselves and not try to be someone that we are not.

It's easier to say than to do. I like to be me, or as the song says, "I Got To Be Me." In fact, I always ask myself, "Why do I want to be someone I'm not?" When I'm myself I can be original. There is only one person I know of who is me, and I feel great being who I am.

I write in my style, I play the drums in my style, and I don't bluff myself into thinking I'm someone I'm not.

All my life I've been that way. I just do what I can do and do it to the best of my ability. It's very easy to do once we know ourselves—who we really are. Acting out my life as someone I'm not is not what would me make me happy.

In the many years I have been in the music world as a drummer I never wanted to sound like GENE KRUPA OR BUDDY RICH. I stayed within my own talents and this was how I wanted to live my life.

I'm also happy that I am not jealous of others in my field. I am so glad that I didn't wish to compete with others. I never tried to be rich and famous. If others thought I had something to contribute in my profession and gave me accolades, that's fine with me. But it's not a good idea to believe your own press clippings. You know the saying: HE'S A LEGEND IN HIS OWN MIND.

I like who I am and I like being myself, not someone else. We each must find out who we are. If we like what we find, then we should stay on the track and follow it until we see what our life brings us. I know I'm happy being me and I like my life the way it is.

I once was asked if I had the chance, would I live my life the same way again? Without hesitation I said yes, definitely. In fact I wouldn't change a thing. I'D DO IT THE SAME WAY AGAIN.

Don't Make Excuses

In my younger days I made all kinds of excuses for things I did that weren't "correct." I had an excuse for anything that I did, that I didn't do, that I should have done. I eventually learned not to do this any longer. I took responsibility for everything I did, RIGHT OR WRONG. This soon became my code of ethics. I felt better off in the long run because I took full responsibility for my actions. I never said someone else was the reason for something I was responsible for.

It was a good feeling and I liked myself better because I had the courage to stand up for my errors and mistakes. If I missed sending out the telephone bill, I took the blame for being neglectful. If I was late, I said I was late because I didn't start out earlier. I didn't blame the traffic or the bus. It was my fault.

While I alone am responsible for my problems I also take credit when I am the one who does the right thing. It took me some years to learn how to stop making excuses. But after I developed this ability to stand up for my own mistakes, as well as my due credit, I really felt very good about myself.

As a professional musician I never made excuses for why I didn't practice and stay on top of my instrument and my development as a professional player. I paid my dues and now at this age I am satisfied with my life, personal and professional.

No excuses. No nonsense. I say yes when I have to say yes and I say no when I mean to say no—NO BULLSHIT.

I think we all have to learn to say yes when we really mean
it and say no when we want to say no.

Take Care of Your Legs

Someone once asked me if there was one most important part of my body that I would take special care of, other than my heart. I answered with ease: I WOULD TAKE SPECIAL CARE OF MY LEGS. I always considered my legs the most important part of my body. Without the use of my legs I would be at the mercy of others. I wouldn't be able to play my drums. I wouldn't be able to transport myself. I would be limited as to what I can do.

Of course, your arms and eyes, ears and heart, stomach and back are all very important. We know that we need all the parts of our bodies to function properly. But for me, my legs are most important.

Pepper Martin, who played second base for the St. Louis Cardinals many years ago, said the way he knew he was finished as a pro baseball player was when his legs were gone. He felt his career was finished when he couldn't run and make a catch in a game. Just think about people with bad legs, who have arthritis and such pain. They can't bend or do many of the things they would need to do in the music world.

So I have concentrated on taking care of my legs. I do squats with weights on my shoulders. I do a lot of bend-overs, leg-ups, and many other exercises that make my legs stronger.

I know that these work because I can still move around and bend over and play my drums. I walk all I want and can dance and reap the values of the many years of training that I have done. I'm certain that stretching, bending, and lifting weights in a steady routine now pays off for me. I think it can pay off for you too—TAKE CARE OF YOUR LEGS; YOU WILL NOT REGRET IT IN THE YEARS TO COME.

Control Your Time

I think one of the problems many of us have is taking each day, 24 hours, and dividing these hours so that we extract something that is valuable to us.

Mentally I break down the day into the following concepts:

- I need to sleep. My sleeping time is about five to seven hours a night.

- I need some time of the day to take care of my personal life. Going to the bathroom, taking a bath (I prefer baths to showers). I need to get dressed and have a light breakfast, lunch and supper. I also need to take my medication for my diabetes. My multivitamin. Of course this doesn't take much time to do, but I must allow for all of it.

- I need time to practice and to write much of the literature that I compose.

- Of course I have a number of pupils and I need time for them. That part of my 24 hours is very organized.

- I also play two, three and sometimes four nights a week with my band.

- I am also involved with a lovely lady and that needs time. I also find time to socialize with friends and family.

I'm very organized in all of these activities. I take care of all of these parts of my day and after doing this for so many years I can control my daily life. For me it works and each of us must make an effort to divide our days so we get to everything that must be done.

I make it sound very simple, but I know it's not easy. Still, I'm certain that your daily life can be brought under your control. All we need to do is apply ourselves and stick with a definite program.

I believe that if we stay on top of an organized system we can control our time. It can be done, and to get the best results, IT MUST BE DONE.

Get Rid of the Drum Study That Doesn't Work

In all areas of study there is material that doesn't work. In my opinion a great deal of the traditional study in drumming doesn't work and I feel drummers should discontinue those areas of study. We should wake up and stop practicing the part of drum instruction that doesn't work and has nothing to do with drum study that has real value in playing drums.

What do I feel should be eliminated? The drummer practices strokes called THE 26 DRUM RUDIMENTS. The word "rudiments," according to the dictionary, means anything in its raw state, the basics, the fundamentals.

This isn't bad in itself. However, these strokes were designed back in the year 1812, before the advent of the drum set as we know it. The drums first took the shape as we know them today back in 1920, when the bass drum pedals were invented. That was the time drummers began to sit at the drum set and use their hands and feet.

The strokes called rudiments were used mostly for the marching drummer, and the music written for the percussion player had nothing to do with the practical art of playing the drums. Thus there isn't any need to study or practice the so-called rudiments, no need to develop the control over this part of drum playing.

Like rudimental strokes, there are some other traditional ideas in drum playing that I feel we should put on the back burner, in order to update the study of our instrument. This is why I feel we should not put serious stress on study that has no value or is not relevant.

I have been called very radical in the study of my instrument. I don't think I am. I feel I am PROGRESSIVE IN THE STUDY OF DRUMS.

So let's give up the study in our field that doesn't work. I might be 80 years old, but I think we should live in these times, not in days gone by.

If It Doesn't Happen Today,
It Will Happen Tomorrow;
If Not Tomorrow, the Next Day

Many times I expected something to happen and it didn't. Then the following day, when I wasn't expecting it, sure enough it happened. What I'm getting at is that I am no longer disappointed when something I expect to happen doesn't happen on the day I was looking forward to it. And if it doesn't happen at all, I don't get depressed, because I figure that's the way it is supposed to be.

Many times I tell my students not to get discouraged or to be hard on themselves. Have patience and ride the days out. You will eventually see that everything turns out all right. Give yourself a chance and keep your spirits and hopes alive.

I know this sounds very idealistic, but I somehow feel that my life has been this way. I never let my hopes die. I've stuck with the feeling that what was to happen for me always does. By keeping my burning hope aflame, everything turned out just perfect. It really did and this is how I've lived my life thus far.

I sometimes feel that there is some special angel looking after me. I very rarely tell someone how I feel about this part of my life. They might think I'm nuts. So I keep these thoughts to myself. I talk to myself many times and tell myself that I always feel SOMEONE OR SOMETHING OR SOME STRANGE POWER IS KEEPING WATCH OVER ME. Like the song says, "Someone to Watch Over Me."

I feel as though someone is looking over me and that my talents and abilities will carry me through the days of my life. No one can tell me otherwise. No outside voice can get through to me and tell me that these silly ideas are just plain nonsense. Where this inner confidence comes from; why I have this gut feeling; how I developed this wonderful attitude about myself — these things have always amazed me.

I felt this way as a young man, even in my early childhood. It became more evident as I grew older. All through my army days. And you want to know something? Here at 80 years old, this feeling is even stronger.

Someone or something is watching and guiding me. It's a great feeling.

If You Don't Know,
Ask Questions of Those Who
You Feel Know the Answer

When I was 13 years old, back in 1933, I started to study with Mr. Aubrey Brooks. He was the instructor at a music school in upper Harlem, here in New York. It was during the Depression, people didn't have much money, and President Franklin D. Roosevelt started the Works Project Administration to get things moving. It was during this time that I started taking drum lessons with Mr. Brooks. Twenty-five cents got me four lessons a month. A lesson a week.

Mr. Brooks was an excellent drum instructor. I was young and really didn't know anything. I knew I wanted to study drums and so this was my best introduction to learning how to play the instrument that fascinated me. Mr. Brooks felt I had some special talents and he took me under his wing.

In school I was a terrible student, but as a drummer I was an "A" student. With my desire and with Mr. Brooks' help I started to learn my instrument.

One of the main things Aubrey Brooks taught me was IF YOU DON'T KNOW SOMETHING, ASK QUESTIONS OF SOMEONE YOU FEEL HAS AN ANSWER FOR YOU. He also taught me to be honest with myself. Mr. Brooks would say, "Learn to say you don't know when you don't know."

And so I say to you: Learn to ask questions. If you don't know something, admit it. Don't feel embarrassed because you don't know something. Otherwise, you'll never get any better. That's why I learned pretty fast, I always asked questions. I eventually got answers to my questions, even if they just led to more questions. I never bluffed when I didn't know something and I needed to understand it better.

I also kept in mind something else Mr. Brooks said: MUSIC IS THE STUDY OF SOUND THROUGH MATH. GET BETTER IN MATH AND YOU WILL BE A BETTER MUSICIAN. Mr. Brooks would also say, "If you can't read music, get a day job."

I remember that in my early days of drum study, I was very poor in math. So I became a good student in math, reading, and drums. I studied very seriously and eventually my math got better and I knew what I was reading. Consequently, my playing got better.

Now that I've been playing almost 68 years, I have grown as a mathematician and, I hope, as a musician. All of this proved to be important in my life, and thanks to Mr. Brooks, these ideas sunk into my thick skull, and I made use of the abilities to read and play music.

Some People Say Practice Makes Perfect — Don't Believe Them

I practice many hours every day and I'm far from pefect. I never met anyone who is perfect, and I never met anyone who even approaches being perfect. I've often thought that if any of us were perfect, we wouldn't be able to get along in this imperfect world of ours.

I think this statement should be amended to INTELLI-GENT PRACTICE WILL GET RESULTS. At least I feel that if we know how to practice we can develop our talents and be the best as we can be. This makes more sense to me. I've searched all my life for methods of practice, and I feel I have an excellent system and get wonderful results from my system of training. I've reached a very high professional level in my music abilities. This may sound like I am bragging. It is not said in a manner that I think I'm the best and no one can be better than I. I just mean that I practice with a very organized program and day-to-day I see marvelous results.

With all the practice I do, I'm still never going to be perfect. I will be able to gain professional abilities and perform to the best of my talents. This allows me to perform as I am capable in the music world. It's sufficient for my satisfaction.

I never strove for perfection. I knew at an early age that I would never be perfect because I couldn't reach perfection. All professional musicians I know and have met eventually realized that they too couldn't reach perfection.

If you are fortunate enough to develop a good, solid practice system, then you will be on the road to success. Of course after you have developed your skills, this doesn't mean you will be able to sell your abilities to those who wish to use you and your talents. This now brings in other talents that you need to work on as a professional. You need to study business. You need to know how to promote your talents so others will wish to use you. You also have to know how to deal with other people. Others have to like you. Others must feel that you are what they need. In short, you need to BELIEVE IN YOURSELF.

Believe in Yourself

You must believe in yourself![1] You must feel you have the ability to do your thing. I believe in myself and I believe I can do anything I want to do. The older I grew, the more I was certain that I had trained myself properly and that I knew my craft and what was required of me to be in my profession. I was convinced that I was skilled enough to play the drums. That I was as good as I could be at the time I was called upon to do a professional job.

That was how I felt years ago and how I still feel. I don't need someone else to tell me that I can do my thing. Each of us should know what our capabilities are, what our limits are, and just how far we can develop our talents.

I know that sometimes we can't judge ourselves and know just what we can and can't do. There are times we have doubts about who we are and to what extent we can take our abilities.

As for myself, I always knew that I could do what I had to do, because I believed in myself. Yet I never fooled myself into thinking I was better than I was. I studied and trained and practiced my tail off. As they say in my business: I paid my dues.

I'm still paying my dues. I wake up every morning and know that I will not get better if I don't stick to the system of study that has brought me to the point I am now.

---

1. My editor told me of a line from Ozzy Osbourne: "You've got to believe in yourself, or no one will believe in you." Now you know I didn't think of that one! But there's a lot of truth to it.

Someone asked me how far I can go as a drummer, even at the age of 80. I said I believe that I can at least hold on to my present talents. I believe that, because I believe in myself.

I believe in myself, as you should believe in yourself. This is most important. I feel as long as I believe in Sam Ulano, I can go on until the body stops.

The Computer Atop Our Shoulders, a.k.a. Our Brain

I don't know how many of you think of the brain in the same way I think about it, but this is how I see it: OUR BRAIN IS OUR COMPUTER ATTACHED TO OUR SHOULDERS. This makes sense to me, and now as I work toward age 81, I see this concept as very appropriate.

Like a computer, I can have total recall from the information I've stored in my brain over the years. I learned how to read music; how to play with all kinds of bands; all styles of music. It's a wonderful device and even more fantastic that I still have control over it. I find it a great part of my life that I still have control over how I think, how I function, and what I do in my profession. My mind is ripe with ideas, day in and day out. What a wonderful feeling!

I tell you now that I learned to develop my abilities and have complete control of my brain. I try not to forget what I studied and to make use of the talents I trained. You'll be happy when you realize this about yourself. Who knows, maybe all the years of learning helped me stave off Alzheimer's disease?

Make plans now in your early life to compile as much knowledge as you can so that you can take advantage of it in your advanced years. Take it from me, you'll be happy that you did.

Listen to Others

All my life I learned how to listen to what others had to say to me. This was important to me because I developed the ability to be a good listener. I learned to make use of what others had to say to me. I still learn from listening to what others have to say. Sometimes someone might say something that sets off an idea that may expand how we think about certain subjects. It's a great approach to living, because none of us has all of life's answers.

People like to know you are a good listener. It shows that you are compassionate and may allow others to want to express themselves to you. As a drum instructor I do lots of talking, but I sometimes find that I must be the listener. OVER THE YEARS I LEARNED HOW TO BE THE ONE WHO KEEPS MY MOUTH SHUT AND MY MIND AND EARS OPEN. I think it's good to be able to listen to others. Sometimes the other person might want to ask questions of you and then take what you say as advice.

Someone once told me listening is a good way to win friends and be a part of other people's lives. I have found this to be true as well.

As you can see, there is much at stake with being a good listener.

No One Can Say What Will Be

I know there are people who believe in fortune-tellers. If you believe this, it is your business. But for me, I think it is all foolishness.

Hard work, hard study, hard practice every day with a system and an instructor who can teach you—I find this to be the answer to our future.

I wrote elsewhere that we must be in charge of our lives. We must believe we can accomplish whatever we wish to do. No tricks or outside person can direct your life by reading cards, your palm or other silly methods. You must study and develop your system for life.

At the age of 80 and working toward 81, I am convinced that we alone can be the master of how we develop our lives, to what level we will develop, and how we can succeed in what we have chosen to do with our lives.

No fortune-teller can come up with an idea as to how we must live. We are born, we develop our education, and as we mature, we know how to follow our dreams and become who and what we wish to be.

I never thought of seeking a reader, some mystic that will tell me how to build my life on their stupid nonsense.

However, if you are someone who has confidence in this form of life and believe that you should follow what they say to you and you want to pay your bucks for this silliness, I say go for it. There is no one who can tell me that they can predict what I must do and tell me what is going to happen to me. I can tell you this with certainty: NO ONE CAN PREDICT MY LIFE FOR ME.

Don't Believe Your Own Press Notices

Sometimes we think we are better than we are. To me this is very dangerous and sometimes it can come back to haunt you. It's great getting good press, but these kinds of notices should not affect how we think about ourselves.

If others wish to write about me and feel I deserve good write-ups, this is all well and good. But I don't allow this notoriety to make me have a different concept of who I am and what I have accomplished. I accept such praise as a reward for what I do in my field, without getting a swelled head or inflated ego.

Being someone you're not can backfire on you and maybe turn people off from wanting to enjoy your abilities. BE YOURSELF AND WHATEVER PRAISE YOU GET PUT ON THE BACK BURNER. Remain natural and be real and don't think you are the greatest. Be a regular guy and people will love you more than you know. I have often found that the better the professional was, the more real that person was.

Keep it simple. Keep it plain. Don't put on any airs. Don't act as if you are the only one in your field. There are others and you should try to be real and not someone you think you are because of someone else's perception of you. Be yourself.

I think this is very important as you go up the ladder and develop your abilities. People will know you and recognize your talents and eventually accept you for who you are.

What Goes Around...

W've all heard the expression, "What goes around, comes around." This means that whatever you do in your life comes back to you. From the good you do, you get back good, and from the bad you send out, you get back bad. I am a big believer in this philosophy—and, yes, payback can be a bitch, but it can also be incredibly rewarding.

I teach drums and I have always tried to train my students as a professional and these students respect this quality in my instruction style. They appreciate the efforts that I put into my teaching style. Many buy my books because they feel my writing is honest and that I try to do my very best. I want my students to be the best, and this attitude comes through in my educational work.

I just celebrated my 80th birthday with a party, and there was such a great outpouring of honest love for me from my pupils. I'm not trying to be a big shot, but there was a wonderful audience from my friends. So I honestly feel that this audience gave me back what I gave out over the years.

I try to give my students my all and to me this is what I want to do as an instructor. I GIVE MY ALL AND I FEEL I GET A LOT MORE BACK FOR WHAT I PUT OUT. Know what I mean?

There of course are some people who are always takers and never givers. Remember that in your life those who you meet are walking advertisements for the type of person that you are. It's your choice whether they're good or bad advertisements.

Dress to Impress

When I was a young fellow, about 17 years old, I joined a musician's union. On Wednesdays, the members would meet at the union hall and exchange stories, and many times other musicians would give each other gigs for the weekend. I made it my business to be at the union hall, but after a few months I found no one paid attention to me and I was never offered a gig.

A good friend of mine lived in the Bronx and we sometimes would take the same train home, since we lived near each other. This particular Wednesday, we both got on the train and discussed the union and Jerry asked me if anyone had given me a weekend gig. I said no and Jerry pointed out to me that I should dress like a professional. A suit and tie. Look like I'm busy. Then maybe someone would offer me a gig.

So the following Wednesday, I did just that: I wore a suit and looked like I was busy, all dressed up.

As I got to the union hall a sax player I knew offered me a weekend job. The same day, two other people gave me jobs for the same weekend. FROM THAT TIME ON, I HAVE DRESSED IN A TIE AND SUIT. Even now, in the year 2001 when I teach, I dress with a tie and suit. The look has become one of my trademarks.

Yes, occasionally I'll wear a nice T-shirt. But most of the time, I wear a suit and a nice tie. I'm glad I do this because I'm ready all the time. I never know who I'm going to meet. Being dressed up means I am always sharp and I like the feeling it gives me.

I tell all my students it is great to be dressed up all the time. In these times young people dress like slobs, even when they go out at night with their gal to a restaurant. I am told this is the style. Nonsense! It tells me people don't know any better.

Dressing up means we have respect for ourselves and for the people we meet. I sometimes find this gives me an edge. I look professional and I like the feeling it gives me. I'm ready for whatever might happen that day.

Most musicians I meet are dressed in a manner that tells me they don't give a darn about how they look and they are saying to me that there isn't any reason to look well and dress like they are proud of who they are and what they think. That's okay with me because I can only take care of myself. I'm not worried about the other guy. That's their business.

Don't Lie to Yourself

In my younger days I had a tendency to lie to myself, and many times I would believe my own lies. But as I got older I started to realize this practice doesn't work, so I made my mind up that I wouldn't hide behind false ideas. I soon got out of the habit of thinking I was doing something beneficial by lying to myself and to others. NO MORE LIES. I have been so happy about no longer telling lies—fibs, half-truths, whatever you call them. If I have nothing to say, I just don't say anything.

I know a lot of what I am writing about sounds almost biblical and has a religious sound to it. Understand I am trying to give you an inner concept of how I have grown up over these many years.

I am certain many of us have come to the same conclusions about their lives and how they want to live. I think it's easier to be real about yourself. It seems to work for me. I am not making myself into a saint. I just feel the truth is the way to go. Being honest with myself has given me a warm feeling about what I do and how I want to live.

I've always felt that WE GET CAUGHT IN OUR OWN TRAP OF SAYING THINGS THAT ARE NOT SO. Eventually this takes away from our real life and who we are.

I have students who tell me how many jobs they are doing and that they are playing with great players and great bands. Then I find out this is not so, and they get embarrassed because the truth has come out. I say to these people, "Don't say what isn't so because it can cause you trouble in the long run."

My Mother Once Said That When We Stop Being a Student We Are Finished

When my mother said this to me I was quite young and really didn't understand what she meant by it. As I grew older and decided what I wanted to do with my life, I started to know what she meant: No matter how good we become in our chosen field, we must always keep learning.

This doesn't necessarily mean we should always be taking lessons from a teacher, but we must always be studying. Doctors do it. All types of "experts" do it (it's how they got to be experts). Even teachers—good ones anyway—remain students all of their lives. So having matured and reached the age of 80, I understand exactly what my mother was saying to me. In my later years, I practice continuously. Study my instrument. Write about my instrument. Read as many different musical journals as possible and make a serious effort to stay on the top of my profession.

I tell all my students that no one else can practice for them. They themselves must do their physical one-on-one practice. They themselves must stay in the best physical shape possible. Watch what they eat. Keep their weight down. Eat what they like, but in moderation. Again, I probably sound very idealistic, but I'm being real.

I talk to myself every day. I say, "Ulano," (that's me)... "Ulano, DO YOUR PROFESSIONAL PRACTICE." I always talk to myself. I tell myself that no one else will do my work for me and no one can practice for me. Sounds nuts to you, reading this, but in reality it is so true. No one can make me better except myself. No one has control over my life but me.

I keep in the back of my mind what Mom said to me: "Always be a student." Never stop learning and never let my talents fall apart. Believe me, this works. I'm like many of you out there in that I like to dream and wish. BUT DREAMS AND WISHES NEVER COME TRUE UNLESS WE MAKE THEM COME TRUE.

And now I pass this on to you. When we stop being a student, we really are finished. Nothing will happen in your life unless you work at making it happen. I'm certain that this becomes much clearer as you get older and start to reach the age where you are "adult" enough to understand this as well as I do now at 80.

Eighty is such a great age if you are in good physical and mental shape. By being a student at all times you will always be improving and always be ready for your success.

I always thank my mom for the profound statement she left with me.

From Our Eyes Down
We Are Just Flesh

Think about this: From our eyes down we are nothing but flesh, and all of that flesh is controlled by our brain. As I said elsewhere, our brain is our computer atop our shoulders. It controls everything we do. Our hands can't think, can't see, can't hear. The brain-computer tells our body how to move and do the actions we do.

Each of us develops and stores information in our brain-computer. Some of us become anything we want to be and others never become anything. They may have certain desires, but they never develop these ideas and so never become anything in their lives. It's too bad because we each can be what we want to be, and be the best at what we are.

All of us have fears that we wouldn't be very good at what we'd like to do and so we never live out what we wished we could be. There are also many of us who are not certain as to what we want out of our lives, and so never reach out and develop our talents.

Once we understand, however, that our brain-computer is where it all starts, we can make sense of these things. ONCE WE DEVELOP THE USE OF OUR BRAIN-COMPUTER, WE START TO KNOW WHO WE ARE AND WHAT WE WANT TO BE AND WHAT WE WANT TO DO WITH OUR LIVES. It is all connected and the body doesn't do anything until the brain-computer tells us that we can do whatever we want to do. This to me is the secret of life!

My brain-computer told me that I could be a professional drummer. I could also play with a band. I also knew I could teach and write about the instrument I love. My brain-computer told me I can sing, direct a band, develop ideas in my profession that others never could do. Or should I say were afraid to do? Maybe we're afraid of what people, particularly in the same profession, would say about us? Who knows why some of us don't develop our talents. Maybe their brain-computer hasn't told them they could be anything they wish to be.

Of course, I've also learned that being what I wanted also means listening to others whose brain-computer has been trained and can explain to us how to use ours. We need professional direction to be what we want to be. Once we find that direction, we need to apply it through hard practice, long hours of review and study, and THINKING DIFFERENTLY. I learned I needed patience as well. When I realized this is what it took—guidance, application, patience—I began to know in my heart that I could do what I wanted to do.

A great musician once said it is so easy when we know how. This is so true. IT IS SO EASY WHEN WE KNOW HOW. Keep in mind that the brain-computer tells the rest of the body what to do. There are no tricks, no shortcuts, no easy ways to do anything in life. Once we have accepted this and have begun applying our mind to those things that really matter, we know the secret of a happy life.

Being Overweight Is Dangerous

I think we can all agree that being overweight is not healthy. It can bring on many of the problems that can be dangerous to our being able to function in our daily lives. There is no question about this.

I speak with some authority. Back in 1960, I weighed 320 pounds. I was up there! And I have experienced the problems being overweight brings. (How about not being able to fit behind a steering wheel?!) The strange thing about that time in my life is that I wasn't really aware of the terrible physical condition I was in. I wasn't sick, I thought, and I can still play and teach and study my instrument. And if it had gone on much longer, I still wouldn't be aware—I'd be dead. Or, at best, struggling.

Earlier I mentioned I was fortunate to be teaching a young chap, Jimmy Roach, who was involved in body conditioning. He brought me to Sigmond Klien's gym and with Sigmond's help I was alerted to my bad body problems. Sigmond hit a button in my brain. I knew I had to do something about myself, and I can honestly say that I WAS SMART ENOUGH TO HEED SIGMOND'S ADVICE. In addition, I had influential friends helping me. A lovely lady by the name of Dorothy Reynolds and a gentleman who owned a big drum shop, Al Wolf, also helped me realize I had to help myself get on the right physical track. (By the way, I fell deeply in love with Dorothy Reynolds, but that's a story for another day…!)

I spent 13 straight years learning how to exercise and train my body. I still do my lifting weights routine, every day, and I never felt better in my life. Yes, it was and still is the right thing to do. It has stood the test of time.

I keep in mind the picture I had of myself when I was 320: I wore a size 54 jacket. A size 52 pants. A size 18 shirt. I look back on that and say I was obscene. It wasn't the best of times for me. I was wearing someone else's clothes. I needed to wake up to the danger of the physical wreck I'd become. Any of you reading this who are out of condition need to look at yourself and catch yourselves before it's too late. You can do it if you become aware of what is in store for you later on down the pike. Once you realize this, and incorporate a simple, effective plan for weight loss, you've got it licked!

If you like being overweight, that's your decision. I don't. And if you don't, then you are able to call the shots and take charge of your life and find the answers to feeling great with yourself again.

Sinatra Once Said Taking Direction Makes a Professional

Some years ago, I was listening to an interview of Frank Sinatra by Bill Williams, a disk jockey (or these days I guess they're called radio personalities or talk show hosts). This was on station WNEW. Bill asked Frank what he thought was the most important quality a person needed to become a top professional.

By the way, the word professional literally means someone who gets paid. It doesn't mean an expert in one's field. However, most of us like to think of being a professional as someone who is the best in their field. I, too, like to think of a true professional as a person is tops, an expert, one of the best at what they do.

Sinatra didn't bat an eye. He said, "It's the ability to take direction." Sinatra said he has a style and is considered a top pro because he can take direction. Direction from the arranger who arranged the tune. Direction from the band leader. The two main musicians at a session. After he takes direction from the arranger and the conductor, Sinatra said, he then can add his style and whatever liberties he might take in singing a certain song. To me that makes so much sense!

Sinatra went on to say that we all must take direction in whatever type of work we do. The bank manager tells everyone what has to be done and how he or she wants things done. The general directs the army. The admiral directs the navy. The coach or manager of a ball club directs the team and calls the shots. IF WE CAN'T TAKE DIRECTION FROM WHOMEVER IS IN CHARGE, WE SOON WILL BE OUT OF A JOB.

Some of us may have a problem with our ability to take direction. But it is a must if we are to become true professionals. Give this some thought and learn to take direction. The ability to take direction, Sinatra said, is the most important quality one must have to be a top professional. I totally agree.

Never Anticipate the Next Day

Live for today…tomorrow, we don't know what to expect. Tomorrow doesn't come for some of us. I know that's a very cold statement. But it's the truth. We may not wake up tomorrow. We just don't know what to expect.

Yet, while you can't anticipate tomorrow, you can prepare for it, so that should it arrive (and there's a very good chance it will) you can live it to the full. That's the best we can do. Study hard, train everyday, and get ready for the challenges ahead. Tomorrow becomes today, so work toward it by making the most of today.

That's how I look at what's in store for us as we travel life day-to-day. I develop my talents and my body so that when tomorrow arrives I can say to myself, "Sam, you are ready for today."

And what happens when you are not ready for today, when you didn't work on things yesterday and don't work on them again today? WE REGRET IT. And that's no way to live. It interferes with life. Tomorrow is a great day to look forward to if you're doing all the things you can today to make it great.

I try to take each day at a time. I try not to live in the past. I try not to build up my hopes for what I would like to happen the next day, and I try not to tell others what I expect to happen the day after today. I do this so that I don't miss out on the only time we have—RIGHT NOW. That way, I simply remain positive and think that good things will develop each day. I tell all my students: Don't jump the gun. Take each day as it comes along.

Don't Hesitate

I wrote earlier that we must make decisions and we must carry them out. Be definite in what you plan to do with your life and develop these decisions you make. Not doing so is like DRIVING YOUR CAR AND SIGNALING THAT YOU ARE GOING RIGHT, THEN GOING LEFT. This can cause a great deal of problems.

Now I say: Don't hesitate.

If you are going forward, don't hesitate in what you are doing. I try to make up my mind to what I am going to do and I do it. Hesitation can be dangerous because it sets up a feeling of indecision with our family, our friends, the people we work with, and especially, with ourselves.

As a musician, I can't hesitate or I'd be doing some other type of work. On nights we have gigs, we start at 7 o'clock and end at 11. In that time, my band knows what I want done. What type of songs we're going to play. I make definite decision as to how the band will perform. At the same time, we are in tune with the audience—they influence what we play as well. If I hesitate I miss that immediacy and the band might not sound as good as we can.

Our sets include swing, dance tunes, some Latin music, some jazz. Music is a world of movement. We play without hesitation. No going right when the song calls for going left. Hesitation leads to indecision, and vice versa. And neither leads to music.

Use All of Your Talents

I'm a big believer that all of us have many talents. The big problem is that some of us don't know it, and so we never develop the talents we have.

For example, I feel I have the talent to play and teach my instrument. I have the talent to write books on the study of drums. I have the ability to play in a band and to play all types of music. I have the talent to sing. I'm not a great singer, but I can sing in tune and can remember the lyrics to quite a few songs. I know my keys. I can sing and play drums in rhythm.

I also have the talent to lecture about my instrument. I can run seminars and answer questions about drumming. I have the ability to publish and advertise the books I write. These are some of the talents I have. I know I have these abilities and can carry out to completion what I set out to do.

I tell all my students to study their talents and train themselves to use the many talents they have. I think it's important we do this because it allows us to function in many areas of our careers and our lives.

Some of us have the talent to work at a bank. To run a company. To teach people. Whatever our talents may be, I feel we should develop all of them, because we're fortunate enough to be born with them.

Of course we must study ourselves and try to discover just what special talents we have. And then we have to develop them. Honing our talents gives us more opportunities to do what we really want to do with our lives. It also ENABLES

US TO BECOME PROFICIENT AT WHAT WE DO so that we can get back what we put in.

I think it's truly a shame that many of us do not improve our talents and, because we don't train everyday, never reach the goals we are after.

I tell my students that they need to investigate what their talents are and study how to use these talents. Of course this doesn't mean we can develop all of our talents. But (and I can only speak from myself here) making a strong attempt at discovering and nurturing my talents has helped me understand myself, which in turn has enabled me to go after what I want. As I matured as a professional drummer, I was able to make use of my multiple talents. I believe we all have a great amount of talent. Check it out for me, would you please, and let me know what you find!

Know Your Good Sides

We live within ourselves. We should know what we are capable of doing. No matter what it might be, I feel we should know this about ourselves. We should know also what we like and don't like. What we can do well and not so well. I always say WE KNOW HOW MUCH MONEY WE HAVE AND HOW MUCH OUR BILLS ARE, SO WHY SHOULDN'T WE KNOW WHO WE ARE INSIDE? It's important to know this about ourselves.

Of course, many of us are afraid to face up to who we are and what our abilities are. We fear what others think about us. We wonder whether other people like us. We worry that we won't make sense of understanding just who we are and what our limits are. Because of these fears—very real, but just fears nonetheless—we may never reach the levels we could if we act on our self-knowledge.

Fear essentially boils down to: WHAT WILL SOMEONE DO TO ME? And do you know the answer? *Nothing.* Absolutely nothing. And it's amazing how fast people forget about you after you do whatever you are doing, particularly on stage. No one is going to kill you. No one will go around the world telling everyone how much you stink. And even if they did, it's your choice to listen to them or not!

Know your strong points. Train them. Use them in your life. I may sound very conceited to you, but I know what I'm good at and I've spent my life developing these points. Now at 80 I'm proud of myself because I now have control of my talents.

Do You Know Who You Are?

It's important that we know who we are. Once we know who we are we then can express and develop ourselves better. I know who I am and where I am at this stage of my life.

As a musician, I know that all my life I have been studying and playing the drums. This allows me to go after my ideas as a musician. I know I can play with a band and perform on stage as part of the band. I know I have the mind of a percussion player, and I know that I have a good ear for hearing and playing the sound of music with other musicians.

I learned that music is the language of sound. As a drummer I play the rhythm in a band, while most of the other instruments play the melody and the harmony. I keep the beat. I feed rhythm into the band and the other players feed off my rhythmic feel. I have learned to anchor the band and hold the band together. When I need it to swing, I swing the band. I also try to add color with my drum playing. I play brushes when I need to hear brush sounds. Playing with a band is a science and I use my sense of who I am to help me perform.

So I know who I am as a musician and where I fit in as someone who plays in a musical setting. Each of us must study who we are. When we do, we can understand who we are. I think it is easy, but that's because I've studied myself. Once we get past our childhood and understanding our talents, WE START TO UNDERSTAND WHERE WE CAN BE PART OF THIS WORLD.

When you know who you are, things become very easy.
When we can progress, we can live the life we want to live.

Once We Find a System of Body Conditioning, We Should Stick With It

Developing a sensible program of training our body and sticking with it provides steady development of our physical system. I have lived with this concept for the past 40 years of my life.

Now I am not involved in the two and three hours a day that many people who do body workouts do. I keep it simple; otherwise I'd have trouble sticking with it. When I wake up I do about 10 to 15 minutes of exercise. Later on in the day I find time to do another 15 minutes. I then do some exercise in the evening.

I know that many of us can't find the time to train ourselves. But I know for a fact that, EVEN WITH A BUSY SCHEDULE, WE CAN DO 15 MINUTES OF EXERCISE IN THE MORNING AND ANOTHER 15 MINUTES BEFORE BEDTIME. The middle of the day is not easy to do. If you can do it as I can, great. But, if not, at least work out in the morning and in the evening.

If you need ideas as to what type of exercise to do, look in the physical fitness magazines and you'll see all kinds of ideas for working yourself into shape. If that doesn't work, go to a gym and get someone who can train you and direct you. As I wrote earlier, that's how I got involved in body development. Get direction. Find somebody who knows and study with a good trainer.

The main idea about all of this is that when you find the right system for you, stick with it. Don't let it get away from you. By now you know my motto: Find a system and keep at it.

We Don't Know Everything

No one knows everything. Some of us know a lot of things, but none of us knows everything. When we think we know everything we are in bad shape. I think that as we get older we learn a lot and we develop our craft and eventually know what our specialty is. It may become a hobby of ours. Or it may develop into the work that we do to earn our living. In that case, our avocation becomes our vocation. Yet we don't know everything, and therefore we never stop learning. WHEN WE THINK WE KNOW A LOT WE FIND THERE IS SO MUCH MORE TO LEARN.

Now that I am 80 I find I am first learning about life, love, sex, marriage, and even my drumming abilities. I have written so many new study books and notice that I haven't even touched the surface of what to write about in my specialty field. I notice that there is so much more I wish to put on paper.

I've been practicing all these years and new ideas pop up in my brain. I am learning new ways to practice. I realize that I must stay flexible, both in mind and in body. So this makes me double my efforts in my daily study and exercise routines.

I am more convinced these days that I don't know it all. I will say I know a great deal about drums and drumming. I will admit that I have developed my talents to a point where I can perform at a high professional level. But this doesn't mean that there is nothing new to develop and study.

By the time we get older, we should have learned something, and that something is that we don't know everything. I only know that I've developed a special program that works for me and for many of my students who study with me. I try to pass on to my pupils reasons why they must constantly practice and learn.

I now know that I know something, but not everything. What's good about this is that it leaves a lot of room to learn as much as I can. That makes it fun for me. I am certain it can be fun for you also.

Don't Be in a Hurry

It takes time to get better. (In my case, at age 80, I must be close to perfect!) Make an honest effort to get better. The more you try, the better you'll get—and the better you get, the more this guiding principle will become a part of your life. I practice every day because I want to be the best I can be. Steady practice means that I have a shot at being just that.

I understand what I must do with my talents. And I know that I must contribute time to my drumming abilities. No one can do it for me; I've already said that once or twice in this book. Life is too short and so I must work at what I can do. If I don't, I may wake up one morning and think that I've let my life slip by. We can't do this to ourselves!

However—and here's the catch—if we rush to do something because we're afraid we're "missing out," chances are we'll do a sloppy job. Then we'll have to do it all over again. In this case, haste truly makes waste: HASTE WASTES OUR PRECIOUS TIME!

It's easy to say, "Don't hurry." But heeding this advice is a common problem for many of us, myself included. We want to get things done so fast that we mess up what should be done clean and clear. (I try to keep that goal in mind: clean and clear.) As in music, you can't rush the beat. Simply put, YOU CAN GET YOUR WORK DONE IN A PROFESSIONAL WAY BY TAKING YOUR TIME. As the song says, "You must remember this: A kiss is still a kiss, as time goes by."

I set aside a program of time to apply to my drum practice. I sometimes want to practice four or five hours. To do this,

I plan it out so that I get all my training time in. I am so happy after I do a solid session that I feel great. You should try to do this too. Take your time and enjoy yourself. Give whatever you are doing your full attention. And don't fool yourself into thinking you can get things done in a hurry. It never pays off.

Have Yourself Checked by a Doctor Once or Twice a Year

I think it is most important that we visit our doctor and get a complete physical check-up regularly. Have our blood checked. Have our heart checked out. Check our eyes. Our hearing. Our weight. Have a colonoscopy (very important). See your family doctor and discuss the need for a complete body check-up if you are to lift weights.

Although this idea seems so fundamentally sound, it's amazing how many people I know tell me they never go to the doctor. To me it's like a musician who doesn't tape himself. How will he know what he sounds like? More important, how will he get better? Catch my drift?

Now that I have reached the good age of 80, I can appreciate the complete body examination. I never let this get away from me. We need this kind of physical check-up.

Over the years doctors have found that I had skin cancer. This was found during a normal check-up! I was operated on shortly thereafter. This operation saved my life. When the doctors discovered I had diabetes, I was given medication to control it.

So I honestly say that GETTING CHECKED OUT BY DOCTORS SAVED MY LIFE. I feel better and now I know how important it is to get checked out. I might not be writing this to you right now if I hadn't.

This precautionary medical check-up also has done a great deal for my confidence—for knowing that my body is in good shape. There is no doubt in my mind that I did the wise thing in having myself looked at.

Check-ups are vital, too, if you're on certain medication. I take the blood thinner Coumadin and every month or so I have a blood test that takes a reading of how well the medicine is working. There is no guesswork about taking this medication. I feel it's better to know what is happening with my blood circulation than to deny that I need medication for a reason.

My suggestion to you is stay on top of what is going on with your body. Remember that you have only one body and we don't get a second one. You can't trade it in like a car. When a doctor says, "This won't hurt one bit," believe him. I think what he or she is really saying is, "If you think this hurts, wait till you see how you feel if I don't do it."

Don't Take Yourself or Anything for Granted

I think we should't take ourselves for granted. We are playing with fire if we take things for granted and think we do not have to be cautious about this attitude. Taking things for granted leads to overconfidence, and in the long run this can backfire on us. (It's backfired on me!)

I tell my students not to let their guard down. We can let things slide by if we're not ready for what may happen or if we feel we don't need to keep working at things. That we do not have to stay on top of our training program—that we've "got it licked" is sometimes an attitude that sets us up for a fall. No one has life licked. We will always make mistakes.

But I can see how it's easy to fall into the trap. Here I am saying we can never be too sure or too certain. So we go around preparing ourselves for the obstacles we may encounter down the road. As a result of our planning, we have some success. But while the best professionals make sure that they are always ready to perform at the best of their abilities, they also know that things can and do go wrong. Knowing that, AND NOT TAKING SUCCESS FOR GRANTED, GIVES US THE BEST CHANCES FOR SUCCESS.

Taking our talents for granted means sometimes we stop training and let our level of quality slide, and just when we need to be at our best we are not at our best. This feeling that we've "got it made" can put us in danger of missing the mark of our top capabilities. Being lax and overconfident tends to make us perform at less than the top of our talents.

You'll be sorry if you take yourself or your talents for granted. This can be a very serious letdown in your career. Pretty soon you start defending the attitude that caused the letdown instead of adjusting it. You don't want this to happen to you, so I say beware, think about yourself, and keep in mind that to feel certain that you need not work as hard any longer is a threat to how good you are or can be. We never should take our life for granted. Be prepared, but guard against overconfidence.

What Would Make You Happy?

Ask yourself this question: What would make you happy? Not what you're thankful for, but what would or does make you truly happy. For me, doing what I want to do, studying and developing my talents, makes me happy.

It's very easy to say what makes me happy because over my years I learned what I like and what makes me happy. I am happy to say that I am happy doing what I do. I love music and my talents have told me that I have the abilities to play and produce music for myself and for the public. When I perform with my band it makes me completely happy. This is the icing on the cake.

It makes me happy to know that I can contribute as well as reap something from all of these years of study. I am certain that doing what we do and getting professional results is what makes us happy. The many hours, years and dollars invested all come together, and the result is a wonderful feeling. All the energy we put in and get back makes us happy.

Think about the work and study a doctor must put in. He or she spends hours in school. Then the doctor spends years in developing his specialties in the medical field. It's very difficult. THEN PEOPLE SAY, OH, DOCTORS MAKE THE BIG BUCKS! But these same people never think of all the things one must give up trying to be a doctor. I always say that whatever a doctor earns after what he's gone through to get it is not enough. I feel the same for people who become teachers in the public schools or colleges. The same for the police and firemen. I recall all the years I had to work on my craft, much less put my life on the line. It's not easy. Then again, who said life was going to be easy?

So following my dreams and desires and working at what I wish to do with my life, which helps me reach my goals, is what makes me happy. I sometimes think it is what makes most of us happy.

Lift Weights Till You're 80
—and Beyond

I give a great amount of attention to lifting light weights as a form of keeping myself in the best physical shape I can. For me, this is the main method I use to stay in wonderful condition.

I must impress on you that, at the age of 80, I feel if I stick with my system of not overeating and of lifting weights, the age of 81 should be one of my best years of my life. How do I plan to be in excellent physical shape and working at age 81? I intend to keep up my body conditioning system of light weightlifting that I have been working on all these years. For me, this system goes back to 1960.

Now keep in mind that no one has promised me that I will be in the best health that I would like to be. In my mind I must work at this.

Some of the other forms of exercise I've tried these past 40 years include running and jumping rope. However, as I got older I felt I had to stop my running program. I began to feel a bit unsteady and, after falling a few times, I felt I wasn't getting the most out of the track routine. I tried judo, karate, and many other body training systems. None of them helped me much.

Yet I always stayed with doing my light weightlifting program—10-pound, 15-pound, 20-pound and 25-pound dumbbells (also called "free weights" because they're not anchored to a larger piece of equipment and you can move them with your hands). My mornings start with a 15-minute lifting program. In those 15 minutes, I lift the 10-, 15- and 20-pound weights. I do leg-ups, body crunches and bend-overs. I start my day this way. I have never felt better in my life than while using free weights. I also find I don't strain myself. I can do my free weights and get a good feeling all over my body.

I supplement the lifting with stretching. The stretching routines I do, the bend-over workouts, help my stomach and back feel wonderful. My neck, my chest, my shoulders, my thighs, calves, and feet all are in marvelous shape.

Remember in the beginning, you do not reap the benefits from the free weightlifting. But as time progresses, little by little, you start to gain strength, flexibility and overall well-being. Day after day the results from this type of body conditioning take shape. It's a great feeling every day.

Here is another encouraging aspect about lifting free weights. Let's say you have been sticking to your lifting program for a few years. And for whatever reason, you stop your lifting system. Let's say you stop free weights for a few years. Then something clicks in your brain that you don't feel as good as when you were in the routine of lifting weights. Something tells you to go back to your program of weight conditioning.

The interesting thing about this is that when you start lifting again, after the first or second week, the body picks up where you left off when you stopped. I found when I stopped running and maybe a year later I started to run again, I had to rebuild my conditioning all over again.

With free weights, the body picks up from where we left off at the time when we stopped. It's one of the great things about body conditioning with weights. Over the years of lifting weights, I noticed this happen a number of times. The body developed muscle tissue and you don't lose muscle. The muscles lie dormant and when you go back to your program of lifting the free weights, the muscles are still there, and in a week or two the body continues on as if we never stopped the weightlifting.

So put that in your brain, and when you get involved with free weights, all you need do is start your program again and build on the previous years that you were lifting.

Another thing about lifting weights is that I stick with free weights (dumbbells) because they're always around. This way, I'm not bound by having to find a "gym" with all its expensive, stationary equipment. I have my dumbbells and they're more than good enough for me to work out with.

Now, you'll notice that there's no "Doctor" in front of my name, and so I have to strongly suggest that you talk to your doctor before you start lifting weights. I also recommend you find a trainer who can teach you to lift correctly. I suggest you buy some of the body fitness magazines on the newsstand and read what the professionals say about body conditioning with free weights, as well. I'm no doctor. I just know what works for me.

Remember Experience Is One
of the Great Teachers

Living through your life is one of the wonderful teachers. From experience you learn through trial and error. Living out the various areas of your life that you are studying is so important. We may be able to get the technical aspects about something through asking questions and reading about the subject. But to develop these ideas, nothing can substitute for real life.

I have often seen the better instructors, no matter what the field is, who have lived through the experiences in their profession. This experience gives the instructor another dimension to him or her. I know that, if a student asks me where, when or how to apply certain parts of the study we do, I can give a deeper explanation of just how to apply the material in a live situation.

As a professional on my instrument and having played in many areas of music, I can write and explain to others how and why to play certain things. It's very helpful to me to be able to take a student through the real life situation of playing with a band.

In my career I have played the wedding scene and shows, with big bands and small groups. I've played classical, jazz, swing, Dixieland, Latin and many ethnic styles of music. Throughout the years I have written a number of study books on all these areas of music performance. I find that, because I have played with all kinds of bands and also as a band leader, I can explain and write about these things with a certain edge—because I've lived through them.

I have also learned how to produce, record, promote, and bring a recording (be it CD, tape or vinyl) to market. I know how to get people to know about the recording and how to get reviews in magazines and newspaper columns. I can then apply this wonderful knowledge life has taught me and show my students ways of developing their career in the music world.

I can give my students reasons and ideas how they can get published and produce their own study books. This opens another method of making an income, so that this student can develop and get into the teaching business.

All of these ideas help a student develop as a professional. Because I have lived through real life's experience, I can show my students how to get into many different things. Then they can go out and get the experience and become a better drummer, teacher, person. Experience is such a marvelous teacher.

Absorbing life's experience is so very important. Getting real life experience along with studying with others who've "been there" is my idea as to how we can be better people.

Tradition Is Nice,
But It Won't Make You Better

To me, tradition is what has happened in the past. It's history and many times it can hold us back from progressing in the times we live in. I said before that if doctors operated on us today as they did 50 years ago, many of us would have died a long time back. Living in the past doesn't help us these days. At least this is how I feel about the past. It's good to know about it, but don't fool yourself into thinking that it's a substitute for working on what needs to be worked on today.

In my field, the traditional study of years gone by does not influence what we do today. The equipment has progressed and has made playing drums easier. (That doesn't mean, however, that the equipment has made us *better*. That's still up to us.) The materials that drums are made of are better. The new sounding cymbals are much nicer. There's better metal for the stands and pedals. Stronger seats to sit on and much improved adjustments of the drums that are superior to what they were in years gone by.

How we study drums is on the move too. But the study books that come out now are still writing about the tradition of the instrument of years gone by. I feel THE TRADITIONAL STUDY OF THE DRUMS HAS HELD STUDENTS BACK and stopped them from being a more proficient player.

I know it's difficult to get drummers to let go of the traditional study, and most educators disagree with my belief. But unless they pay attention to what people like myself are saying, today's percussion students will end up spending many years working on material that will not help them. A good drummer, one who can earn a living at his craft, needs to be as up-to-date as possible.

I guess it's hard to let go of old habits, and since change is hard to come by, this problem will always exist. I'm just saying that simply because it happened many years ago doesn't mean that those bygone methods are still valid in modern times. Tradition may be beautiful, but it is not the key to improving our talents.

Keep Your Professional Life Separate From Your Personal Life

Here is something to think about: Approach your personal and your professional life the same way, but don't mix the two. I say this because what works in making a successful career also works in making a happy home. But when the two come into contact, one area begins to infringe on the other and, invariably, we don't get the most out of either. Let me give you an example of what I mean.

We study to develop our way of making an income so we can make the dollars we need to pay for our personal life. Once we have our professional life developed and we know what we can do to make the bucks we need to exist, we are on the track of being happy with our life. In my case I am a professional drummer. I cover as many areas in my field as I can and this allows me to be active as a professional.

As a professional musician, educator, writer, and lecturer, I don't let my home life disrupt my playing abilities. I must practice every day. I must teach and write new material. Since I have the know-how to do all these parts of my professional life, I take care that I keep myself in the best physical shape and mental condition. I let no outside problems interfere with my abilities. I do not say, I'll practice later or tomorrow. I don't procrastinate. I don't put off today and think I'll get to it the next day or the next week.

I handle my personal life the same way. When I go out with my lady friend and go to a show or just watch TV, I want to enjoy that part of my life. When I am out of my studio I don't think about working. I don't wish I was practicing. I don't allow my personal world to be affected by my professional world. In other words, I work as hard on my personal life as on my professional life. IT MOTIVATES ME TO KNOW THAT I'LL ENJOY MY PERSONAL LIFE MORE IF I TAKE CARE OF MY PROFESSIONAL LIFE, AND VICE VERSA.

If you are married, in love with a guy or gal, and have spent most of your life developing your talents so that you can earn a living, it is important that you keep these two areas of your life separated. It's the only way I've found to get the most out of both.

I Never Saw a Fat Race Horse

Throughout this collection of my philosophy of life, I have written a number of pages dealing with staying in the best physical shape that we possibly can. I always knew that if I stayed in good health, I had a better chance to grow old gracefully. It's true because I noticed that if I keep my steady routine of body conditioning and eating habits, I am able to handle my music career. It's a wonderful feeling to know that I have this part of my life working.

I find that keeping myself trim and not letting my weight get out of control is what makes everything else work for me. I never saw a fat race horse or a fat runner. If you can stay in condition, I know it will make you feel that life can be beautiful.

The trick is to stick to your discipline and stay on course and not allow yourself to fall out of shape, which is easy to do. It's easy to overeat and gain extra weight and so difficult to lose that excess.

We need to FIND A PURPOSE IN ORDER TO STAY ON TOP OF OUR LIVES and make sure we don't lose this control. So when I say I never saw a fat race horse or a fat runner, I use these examples in my mind to know that I must keep myself in the best physical shape, if I am to live longer and be able to play my instrument.

I feel I have to stick with the commitment that goes with caring for my body. You also have a body and you too must dedicate yourself to being on top of it. Only then will you get the results that you want from your efforts.

Ideas on How to Handle Boredom

As busy as I am with teaching, writing and playing professionally with my band, I also experience periods of boredom with my life. Why does it happen to me? This is something I have thought a great deal about and this is how I undo the problem.

I find when I am bored, I try to get to the root of the problem. What do I do? Why—when I feel that I have a lot of talent and ambition—does this empty feeling seem to fill my hours? I say to myself, "Self, why are you feeling this way? What is it that makes a certain amount of my time so nothing?"

These are good questions that I ask myself, so I take time to undo this feeling that comes every so often. Now realize that I find this very strange because I have so many great things to do with my time.

I practice my drums a few hours a day; I also play a few nights a week with my band at the famed Red Blazer Hideaway Supper Club. I have a program of body conditioning that I stick with every day. I do this everyday because I can't allow myself to let my body to deteriorate, get out of shape. You'll recall I said I am now 80 years old (and working towards 81) and that I promised myself that I will try to stay in the best physical shape that I possibly can. Then I have a personal life: I listen to the news, read the newspapers and go to the movies. I also like to go out to dinner, spend time with people I love. I have sisters and brothers that I love and I enjoy getting together with them every so often.

There is so much going on in my life and yet I get these spells of boredom. However, I've come to the conclusion that THIS IS NORMAL AND THIS FEELING EVENTUALLY PASSES. I don't worry about feeling bored or useless. I'm not certain, but I know this is a normal feeling that many of us experience. I just preoccupy my time with my daily tasks and just let it ride until the feeling of being bored goes away.

When I realize that I am not the only one who has this inner feeling of boredom, I feel that I am not alone. My answer for myself is that this is something that comes around every so often, and I have learned to accept this emotion. I try to keep myself occupied or sleep it off and say to myself that maybe the feeling will go away the next day when I wake up. If it doesn't go away the next day, I ride it out and eventually I find that I'm not bored any longer and am back to feeling good about what I love to do.

I sleep it off. I talk to myself and see if I can come up with some method of clearing my mind of this problem. Somehow I get it out of my system and it's nice when it goes away. Amen!

How I Handle Defeat

I am certain that many of us have had to face up to the problem of defeat. Losing isn't easy but we must have some ideas about how to handle defeat. Being a good loser isn't easy. We have to accept that this is the way it is. Whether it's sports, cards, love, business, competition in the arts, friendships, whatever. We must face up to the fact: Someone wins and someone loses. And we're on both sides often enough.

One of my students asked me how I handle defeat. What do I do? How does the situation affect my life, my insides? What goes through my mind when I'm "the loser?" What do I think of so that I can be a person who understands that we all can't be the winner?

The way I approach losing in most areas of life—and perhaps this is a naïve view of the world—is I simply tell myself that maybe next time I'll win. I have to tell myself this is the way it is and I must be a good sport. Otherwise it festers. Besides, I know rationally that I can't win all the time. So in my mind and heart I go with the flow. Life goes on and all I can do is work harder and look forward to winning the next time. If not, then I look ahead and keep trying to improve myself, so that I may be a winner the next time around. It's the only control we have over the situation.

Losing in love is harder, however. I have experienced this and have tried telling myself that I can't go to pieces—that "what is to be is to be." I know the feeling of loving someone so much and then losing them. I've had people I love die or we've broken up and gone our separate ways. Sometimes I don't get over it right away, but I'm strong enough to handle this very serious emotion of love, and I accept that losing out in love is part of the risk. But without the risk, there's no reward.

I feel that in our lifetime we will experience many different stages of love, sadness, happiness, success and losses. We must be strong and accept all of these problems and joys of our lives. IT'S WHAT I CALL GROWING PAINS. Now at 80 and going on 81, I have "grown" a lot! I try to be objective and understand this is what life is about. I am no different than the next person and this is how life is.

When we were born, no one gave us a plan on how our lives will be. We must learn to take the good with the bad. Some defeats are worse than others. Each of us must judge what we want out of our lives, and, as I say, we have to go for it.

As a professional drummer, I have had times when I felt I was the person that should have been given a certain opportunity. But I am happy that someone else got the opportunity. I never call a defeat a defeat. I say that there is a way that it is supposed to be and there are ways that it's not supposed to be. I tell myself to live with it and go on to the next day because something better may await me there.

Happiness

When I was a youngster going to public elementary school, I had no direction each day. I had not yet found what I love to do. I come from a large family. Ten children, a mother and father. And I have a twin brother.

I really didn't like school. I didn't enjoy studying. I was not a good student. I never did my homework. I managed just to get through the days in school and always looked forward to the weekends and holidays. Nothing exciting was happening for me. It was that way through my early days.

I guess my life really started when I was 13 years old. My good friend Harry Kopleman, who lived in my building in the Bronx, got involved with drumming. He saved money and bought a set of drums at Manny's on 48th Street in Manhattan (the same Manny's that's there today). Harry invited me up to his apartment. I was fascinated by this beautiful, mother-of-pearl drum set. It was known as—get this—THE SLINGERLAND RADIO KING GENE KRUPA MODEL. Gene was the drummer with The Benny Goodman Band.

Wow, what a kick! I just was so impressed with beating the skins, as they say. Harry was taking drum lessons from a gentleman named Jules Wishecs who lived on the ground floor of our building. It was the Depression and so money was scarce. Harry paid 35 cents for each lesson. I was invited to sit-in on one of Harry's drum sessions, and I asked his teacher if he would teach both of us at the same time. I also paid 35 cents that I scrounged up by doing little odds and ends for my brothers and sisters and my mom.

I would spend many hours practicing on a rubber drum block. (Drummers use these rubber blocks so the noise doesn't disturb people around us.) I bought my first drum book, also at Manny's, for 90 cents. It was called the Harry Bower System for Drums. And that is how I got started on the drums.

At James Monroe High School, also in the Bronx, the teachers there thought I had a talent for music, so I was made a member of the band and orchestra. It was easy for me because I could read drum music.

Because I found something I loved to do, it affected my schoolwork. I became a good student! I would have to say that drum study was the catalyst that set me off. It made a difference in my life, and I can honestly say as I reflect back on this time of my young life that I'd found true happiness.

To find happiness, you must find what makes you happy and what you love and what can occupy your time. Something that makes you think and feel good. Once you find what you enjoy, happiness is the reward you get back.

Success

What is success to you? Is it making a lot of money? Is it being the best in your field? Is it everybody saying you're the greatest?

To me success is doing something I love and the feeling that my life is beautiful and I'm doing something I want to do. I make enough money so I can live nicely, take care of my family, and keep on doing what makes me happy.

Success to me means that I'm healthy and able to get up everyday and enjoy the things I love. Success means having someone in my life that enjoys being with me. Success to me means people in my field of endeavor like what I do and use my talents because they think I'm good at what I do.

Success to me means that I can enjoy the beauty of each day without having any major hang-ups or regrets. I've reached a point of my life where I feel I've been successful in my chosen field. I still have fairly good eyesight. My hearing still allows me to play with my band. My body is in pretty good condition for someone over 80. My legs are in tip-top shape. (As you know, once your legs start to give you trouble, so that getting from point A to point B is a problem, you know you have serious problems. My body exercise program that I am now doing for forty years, has been the reason that I can boast about my excellent leg condition.)

I feel money is important to live, obviously. We need it to pay the rent and bills, to buy food and clothes, and for our family and for ourselves to enjoy many of the things we like. We need money, there is no denying this. But I don't say it is the most important quality where success is involved. We must love what we do in life. We can't just like what we do, but love it. Working on this aspect of my life, making it come true, this is what success is to me. I love what I do and so I love life.

And that is how I judge success.

All of Us Must
Take Care of Ourselves

After all these years I have come to the following conclusion—that as we get older, we each must take care of ourselves. As a youngster, our parents and others in authority try to bring us up so we can grow into responsible adults. Although we might not have realized it at the time, what they were really teaching us was to take care of ourselves, because nobody would do it for us, no matter how much we wished they would.

We eventually have to learn how to read and write. We understand what the value of money is. We learn how we are to support ourselves and eventually to take care of our family. Our children must grow up as well (though sometimes we forget this). All of us, no matter who, must do for ourselves. If we don't, we'll have trouble being in this world of ours.

This is important, and unless we do this, we will not be able to function in this society. This is how I see it, and I'm certain that all people all over the world understand the same thing. It is an ongoing system for all humans. Sometimes it takes a long time to train ourselves and our families. Basically, what I'm saying is that each of us must develop the three important ideas I described in the early part of this work—OUR HEALTH, OUR EDUCATION, OUR FINANCES. Without these, I say to you, good luck surviving, much less thriving.

My Music Is My Philosophy

I finished the first 54 pages of this book and the next thing you know my computer-brain came up with many new ideas for my philosophy of life. Why this happens to me, I'll never know. But the mind is a very funny thing and works in strange ways. Before you know it there comes another series of ideas and I'm off writing some more of my thoughts. For starters, what is 'philosophy' anyway? I've been told it is how we live and love life. If that's the case, I sure do have a philosophy about life!

Some of us believe in ourselves. Some of us think we are better than the next person. We might not be sure, but eventually we learn about ourselves, what we can and can't do. We never know what will fill up our lives. As for me, I found music. It was food and music that made me happy and still make me happy (though I've come to realize that too much food does not make anyone happy!). BUT MUSIC, SWEET MUSIC…I NEED MUSIC TO MAKE ME FEEL LIKE SOMEBODY.

I once heard someone say that a person without music in their life is a walking zombie. I'm not certain that all of us need music, but I feel music can do so much for us. It makes us want to dance and it makes us happy and makes us laugh and sometimes makes us sad. I know one thing— MUSIC REACHES INTO OUR HEARTS AND MINDS. It touches all of our emotions and then brings about many different effects in our lives.

A movie without background music is boring. A dance without music seems dull. When we hear a symphonic orchestra, we come alive. It gets our attention and makes

us reach higher levels. Music allows us to express ourselves in many different ways.

Just think of the great music written by the great com-
posers: Beethoven, Bach, Mozart. Then there are Gershwin,
Berlin, Rogers and Hart, Mancini, Duke Ellinqton, Jerome
Kearn, Lennon and McCartney, and on and on. Think of
the various changes in early music—ragtime, Dixieland,
swing, be bop, rock n' roll, Latin, rap. Each of these wonderful worlds of sound makes us come alive. Music can
make us live better; it can even help us sleep better!

Many times music gives us something or someone to
remember. We become romantic and may love someone so
much that we might even go to the end of the world for
that person. Prince Edward gave up his crown for the lady
he loved. Who knows what music was behind his decision!
To love someone so much that you give up everything else
in life. Very interesting. Very musical.

Everyone Younger Will Get Older

No one gets younger. However, WE CAN DEVELOP SOME LIFESTYLES AND FIND OURSELVES GETTING BETTER AS WE GET OLDER AND STAYING STRONG IN OUR MINDS. We can develop great habits and interesting concepts about how we want to live our lives. We find many new ways and ideas that get us to accomplish our goals.

If you go back to the early part of this philosophy of my life you read how important I feel about developing a system as we progress in our lives. As the years go on, I am more convinced about this and impress upon you that this is one of the great keys that can bring us to the many things we want. My system is one of priorities: health first, education second, and finances third. I can bet that many of you will come to this same conclusion.

Something that happened to me yesterday may illustrate what I mean…

Yesterday at 5 o'clock I went to the post office to mail a few items. As I was coming back to my studio where I teach and practice, I started to feel very woozy and my head was spinning and all of a sudden I felt myself weaving and bending, and THE NEXT THING I KNEW, I TOPPLED OVER AND FELL INTO A SNOW BANK. There was a heavy snowfall just before the New Year.

Down I went, flat on my back. Immediately, so many nice people were concerned if I was all right. I said I was dizzy and before you knew it three or four people pulled out their cell phones and called 911. In less than five minutes a fire department ambulance came to my rescue.

They brought me to the Veterans Hospital on 23rd Street, and the doctors in the emergency ward took care of me. I stayed overnight and, after having gotten a clean bill of health, I'M OKAY AND BACK AT MY STUDIO WRITING MY BOOK.

I am always impressed with the system they have at the hospital. They take your temperature, check your blood pressure, take blood. They ask what happened and document everything that you tell them. Fortunately, I am a regular patient at the VA, and my complete records are in their computers. This makes it easy for all the medical people to find my medical history.

Developing a system as well as knowing yourself and knowing that each of us changes as we get older are so very important. They have such an exacting system at the VA that it literally saves lives. This is why I feel systems are important, and we can become better people because of them, no matter how young or old we are.

America Is the Greatest Country in the World

I have said the following many times to many people: Had I been born in any other country, I might not have done the things in my field that I have accomplished these many years. I really believe this. Being in America, I was able to write, create and learn my craft. I live in New York City and was brought up here. The challenges in America are outnumbered only by the opportunities it offers.

Because of this opportunity, I have had a large variety of students. As I trained these pupils, I also was training and developing my own talents—as an instructor and as a professional player in the music world. I was able to hear live bands and grew up with all these musical wonders around me.

As I got older, I was able to go out and listen to the best in my field—Buddy Rich, Gene Krupa, Max Roach, Louie Bellson, Art Blakley, Philly Joe Jones, Papa Joe Jones. All the big bands in the day when big bands flourished. I saw and played vaudeville. I played in various summer resorts. I was able to study with a large variety of educators in my field. I was able to develop all my skills as a percussionist. I spent hours of my life practicing and learning from all these influences.

The great thing about all of this is that NO ONE STOPPED ME. NO ONE SAID I HAD TO ANSWER TO THE GOVERNMENT, FOR INSTANCE. I WAS NOT RESTRICTED IN ANY WAY. I HAD TRUE FREEDOM TO FOLLOW MY DESIRES AND DREAMS. As long as I didn't bother someone else, as long as I did my thing, I was free to develop my craft. This was because I was born here in America and lived in this marvelous place, the only place on earth where I was left to my own desires. My family was well aware of this too, and they encouraged me. My mother and father and brothers and sisters also could follow their dreams, as well. Whatever those dreams were.

I know there are people who are dissatisfied with their lives here. To these people, I say go find a place where you would be happier and do what you want. I do not know of such a place. Developing our talents and reaching our desired goals depend on each of us. Wishes are great, but we can't live on wishes. To make wishes and dreams come true we must be realists and live in the real world. No fantasy.

Yes, in my mind, America is truly the place where we can get what we want, but being here alone is not enough. We must work at whatever we want to gain. WHILE THERE ARE LOTS OF OPPORTUNITIES, REMEMBER THAT THERE ARE NO GUARANTEES.

The Best Part of My Life
Was Spending Four Years
in the U.S. Army Band

I have been asked many times about what part of my 80 years were the most important and why?

Let me see if I can answer this for you. On November 6th, 1942, I was drafted into the United States Army. I was 22. I had no idea what to expect. I had no idea where I was going, what I would be called upon to do. No conception of what was going to happen to me, how long I would have to serve, or what was expected of me. I went because I was drafted, like so many young fellows around my age.

Now that I look back on this phase of my life, I have come to the conclusion that these four years were the four most important years of my entire life. Let me explain...

I was an ordinary young fellow, involved in playing the drums. I was already teaching at that young age. I guess I had the ability to explain and demonstrate the study of drumming. Now, mind you, I had only 10 years of drum experience, but I was a very serious student and loved music and drums. I guess it was in my blood.

Anyway, I was inducted into the army at Fort Dix, New Jersey, and was assigned to the 391st infantry band at Camp Breckenridge, Kentucky. It wasn't until I actually arrived at Camp Breckenridge that I realized I was in a band. I was ecstatic. I was so happy that it couldn't have worked out better for me.

In the four years that followed, I gained some of my most important experience as a musician. AS A BAND PLAYER

IN ALL KINDS OF MUSIC SITUATIONS, I PLAYED
SHOWS FOR THE TROOPS WITH BOB HOPE, JACK
BENNY, BETTY HUTTON, JERRY COLONA, AND MOST
OF THE OTHER HEADLINERS THAT WORKED WITH
THE USO. The USO was an organization that sent all kinds
of entertainers to perform for the soldiers just behind the
lines on the battlefields. It was an important part of keep-
ing the morale of the troops high.

During those years, I learned how little I really knew about
life. Living with other people, taking orders, and playing
with accomplished musicians, I learned a lot—and fast.
They made me a sergeant and so I had to learn how to handle other people. IN FACT, I HAD NO CHOICE: THEY
PUT ME IN CHARGE OF A 100-PIECE MARCHING
DRUM CORPS!

I learned so many things in those four years that it's hard
to know where to begin. I learned about my body and how
to take care of it. I learned how to live away from home. I
learned a great deal about reading and applying music in
a big swing band. I was fortunate to have one of the great
sax players in the band who taught me much about playing in this musical setting. Phil Bodner was his name. He
still is alive, as far as I know. He taught me a great deal
about how to take direction and how to play different
styles of music. I was a fast learner, and Bodner was a wonderful bandleader. So the four years were like going to
music college. In fact, it was better than music college
because we were living real life. Hell, I even learned how
to write letters home!

These four years helped me get my drumming together,
and I knew then and there that I needed to learn a great
deal more if I was to become a professional musician.

And so, after the initial shock wore off, I embarked on a

learning odyssey that continues to this day. I began learning about how to be an educator. How to handle students and people. I learned how poor my education was. Little by little, I learned about and corrected my weaknesses. It was a great education. There were things that could have been better, obviously—WE WERE AT WAR AND A GREAT MANY YOUNG MEN DIDN'T MAKE IT BACK. BUT ON THE WHOLE, I DID WHAT I COULD, WHICH MEANT I LEARNED AND APPLIED AS MUCH AS I COULD.

I also saw places I would never have seen. I was in Hawaii. I was in Japan. I traveled throughout the United States. So much to see and so much to do and learn about living and how to handle life's endless challenges. This education has stood me in fine stead. I learned much that I couldn't learn being at home.

As I reflect on these years of my life, I must say they were four of the most valuable years of my growing days, and I will always cherish them. I wouldn't trade them for anything in the world.

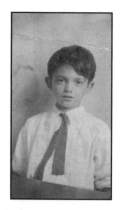

Sam at age 6 or 7

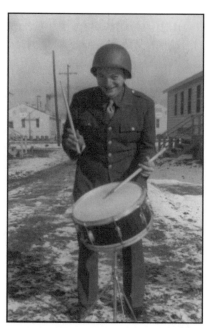

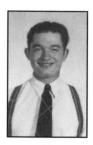

Smilin' Sam, 20 years old

The Army Years, circa 1942

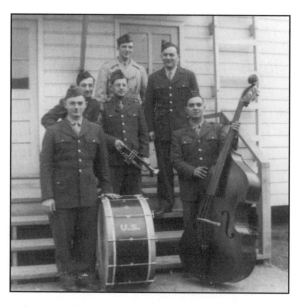

Sam and the Camp Dixieland Jazz Band

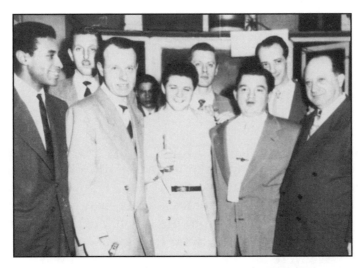

Sam and the 'Gang' in 1952, from left-front:
Max Roach, George Herman (r), Phil Grant, Charlie Perry,
Jim Chapin (r), Sam Ulano, Raymond Suskind (r), Erving Torgman

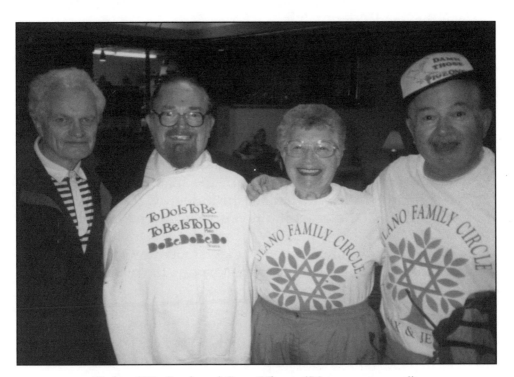

Twins 2X: Saul and Sam Ulano (81 years young!),
Sarah Ulano and Ben Ulanoff (84 years – younger!)

Never Been Drunk
and Don't Plan To Be

I have never been drunk. I knew in my early years that I didn't enjoy drinking. In fact I didn't like being around people who drank too much. I knew that this wasn't for me. I guess it goes all the way back to my younger days when I got into the music business. I saw a very good friend of mine, who had gone to high school with me. We were playing in a summer resort. I was 16 and he was 17 or 18, and I saw him in a band and he was quite discombobulated. All messed up. Then I noticed another of my friends, also an old classmate, a sax player who was so drunk that when he got off stage he was throwing up all over the bandstand.

I said to myself, IF THAT IS WHAT BEING DRUNK IS LIKE, YOU CAN KEEP IT. I made up my mind I wasn't ever going to drink or even try a drink when I play with a band. Then, as I thought about it, I realized I'd never seen anybody function well on booze. So I stayed away from drinking, both socially and professionally. You wouldn't want to be driven by a drunken bus driver or fly on a plane with a drunken pilot, would you? Too many people get into serious trouble when under the influence. It's just not good and is not the best condition in which to perform.

In all my years in music I never understood how someone can think they are at their best when having too many vodkas, scotches, martinis or whatever.

In addition, many people in later years suffer problems from drinking. They do damage to their bodies. They have to pay the price for not taking care of themselves.

I always tell people if they poured 10 gallons of water in their gas tank, they would see the damage they will do to their car. Water doesn't belong in your gas tank, and your car lets you know it, just like your body lets you know that alcohol doesn't belong in it.

Your sense of balance, your judgment, and your thinking process get affected from too much drinking. The body wasn't built to disrupt it with drinking. If you are under the impression that drinking will be good for you, think again. However, I always say "to each his own" and if this makes you happy, go to it. You'll see that drinking is dangerous for your health. Take it from me.

Some Important Things I've Learned

I was once told that by the time we get older, we should have learned what works and what doesn't work. We should know what is important to us and how to correct the mistakes we have made so we don't repeat them again. I'm sure many of you reading this book have looked back at your own life and remembered things that you did and never want to repeat, and other things that work for you and that you continue to take joy in. Here are some of my conclusions that I have come to realize.

- The first important thing I learned over all these years is to make sure I stick to my body conditioning routine. This has stayed uppermost in my brain. I wake up and do my muscle stretching and strengthening routine. I make every effort to do this when I wake up. I have learned that at 80 this has been the best thing I've done for my well-being. It works and I intend to continue this until I die.

- The next thing I've learned at age 80 is that the musical talents I have developed must continue to be developed every day of my life. By working at my craft, practicing and studying, I will always stay on top of my percussion abilities. Like the Boy Scouts and the Marines—I will always be ready. I would be very disappointed in myself if I allowed myself and my skills to deteriorate. I would never forgive myself. Besides, I make a living playing my drums and I love playing this musical instrument. It fascinates me and gives me great pleasure.

- Another thing I have learned at 80 is that worry doesn't solve any of my problems. So I don't worry about what will be. As I say, I like to take care of business and things will work out. There is no need to worry. Many people I know always worry and this never helped them fix what they are worried about.

- I also learned that we come into this world and only live once. After we are gone, we don't get a second chance, and so I feel that while I am here I must try to do the best I can do. I try to stay out of trouble. I don't do what I don't need to do. I do the best that I can. I'm not trying to be perfect, and I do not let my ego get the best of me. I am who I am and that's all I can be, nothing else.

- Finally, I learned something a long time ago that I still live by: MY MOTHER ONCE TOLD ME THAT EVERY DAY YOU WAKE UP YOU SHOULD HAVE A GOOD TIME WITH YOUR LIFE. Of course, I have to take her advice and I try my best to enjoy every living hour of my life. It's easy to do if you don't allow unimportant things to get in your way. My mom was a smart lady, and she knew what she was talking about.

I Don't Give Opinions on Things
I Don't Know About

What I don't know about, I try not to give my opinions on. Some things I put in this category include politics, medicine, what it's like to be at a place I never visited, and legal matters. I feel that I can't give an opinion about something in which I am not trained.

My favorite line is, "How can you talk about something that you are not experienced in?" I don't think you can. I know I can't give my thoughts on what I don't know about. I'll ask questions instead. I'll listen to people who I feel know about the subject and that's the best I can do. Now, when I talk about music, the profession or its study, we are in my ballpark, and this where my experience lies. I can talk about this subject because it is my thing.

This is one of the reasons why, when I was operated on for three herniated discs in my spine, I never looked for a second opinion—one that was closer to my own thinking, which was simply that I, like the next guy, don't want to get cut open. Similarly, when the doctors at the Veterans Hospital said I had skin cancer and needed an operation right away, I didn't question them. The operation was done immediately.

When I was told by the doctors I had diabetes, I didn't question it. I JUST ASKED WHAT I COULD DO TO CONTROL IT? THEY TOLD ME WHAT TO DO AND I HAVE FOLLOWED THEIR INSTRUCTIONS FROM DAY ONE. The reason I didn't question them is because I am not a doctor and I had to trust these people and put myself in their hands. I'm glad I did. I am healthy today because I listened to the medical people and took their advice and direction.

I know so many friends of mine who are dead today because they didn't take the medical advice given to them and kept getting other opinions. That was the end of them. Sad.

Let me put it this way: When I need carpentry work done, I find a carpenter. I go to a dentist to tell me what to do about my teeth. An eye doctor to take care of my eyes. An audiologist to take care of my ears and hearing. I let a podiatrist take care of my feet. A cardiologist takes care of my heart, and so on. If you haven't learned this in your younger life, you will have trouble later on.

What I don't know about, I keep my mouth shut and let the people who know direct me and tell me what must be done and how it is done. It's amazing how well everything in my 80 years of life have worked out. Sy Oliver, famous bandleader, arranger and musician, once said to me: "Sam, it is so easy when you know how." Amen.

I'm Curious About the Methods Employed in Other Fields of Endeavor

I was always interested in the methods used to develop other fields, not only in music. How did someone get involved in the post office or the police department? One of my students works for Citicorp Bank. His expertise is in estate planning for senior citizens. I found it interesting what he told me. He studied finance in college and now he makes good money and is only 34 years old. He has been studying with me for 22 years and is a wonderful drummer and can read fly paper. A wonderful talent who really knows his business—both of them.

Every field of endeavor has its unique systems for study, and I am fascinated by these methods and how they are used, how they are studied, how they're taught. It has always been interesting to me. The reason I am interested in these methods is that sometimes there are ideas I can use in my field of music.

I have studied with a lot of teachers in music over the many years I have been in music. I have studied trumpet, piano, guitar, bass, timpani, vibes and a number of other instruments. I was curious about the methods these teachers used. Some of the methods were good and some were not so good.

I teach a number of melody players who have problems in breaking down rhythmic studies. I try to explain how drummers read and use the written sheet to help them understand the overall picture when the arranger writes the drum chart. What the arranger is trying to convey to the drum player.

I am glad that I did study these ideas and methods and, along the way in my life, have understood what others have done. Thus, the study of methods from all people I meet, and why and how they study, and the system they use to develop their abilities in their particular field have always been valuable to me.

There Is Nothing
to Be Nervous About

I tell all my students that no one is going to arrest you if you goof up. There isn't anyone who says that when you make an error or a mistake or mess up in a live performance you're going to be murdered, arrested or ostracized from society.

As for me, I can't remember when I was nervous and worried about my performance. Maybe there is something wrong with me. Maybe I'm too dumb and don't know any better.

Remember none of us are infallible. We all can stumble and get the jitters. I never thought there was anything I should fall apart about. I TRY TO DO MY BEST AND BECAUSE I KNOW MY CRAFT, I FEEL CONFIDENT THAT I CAN CONTROL MY NERVOUS SYSTEM. I can be under the greatest pressure, and it will not make me lose my balance.

I think many of us that are frightened and suffer stage fright have not been trained well. Really knowing what to do on stage or at an interview for a new job, or whatever the situation might be, should teach us to have control over ourselves.

Of course, most of us are worried about what people will think of us. In school or even at home at a young age, a teacher or person in authority might have scared us and we didn't know how to handle it. Then there are those times when we meet a lady or a lad and fall in love. We may be confronted with some serious part of our lives. Perhaps getting married. Meeting a future mother- or father-in-law. This could be scary.

It's fear that upsets us. But we need to remember what President Franklin Roosevelt said: "The only thing we have to fear is fear itself." How true. Just see it for what it is. Feel it, but then put it in perspective. Control it; don't let it control you.

I have often told my students they must have a strong belief in their abilities. There should be no negative thoughts in their minds. Study yourself and learn as much about yourself as you can. What upsets you? What thoughts enter your mind when performing? Discuss these things with yourself, and, remember, no one is going to harm you. The greatest achievements have been made in the face of fear, once that fear is revealed and put in perspective.

Be Prepared

I know I might sound like a broken record (no pun intended), but throughout my life I've always tried to be ready for anything, particularly my next gig. Preparation is my motto. And so I try to be ready in my talents, with my equipment, the clothing I need, knowing the directions of where to go, who I am working for, his or her phone number, what the occasion is at which I will be performing. Whatever the details are, I find that you actually get less bogged down in them the more you understand them.

I'm not worried what the next person is doing. Male or female. They must get themselves ready and they must be prepared for what may come. Like they say, we can't predict the future and we can't know what to expect. We have a sketch in our minds as to what may be, but this only unfolds when we are in the live situation. So be as prepared as you can for any situation.

Being ready makes my mind comfortable because I know I am well-prepared, and when I get to the live performance this PREPARATION HELPS MY CONFIDENCE. I'm much more sure of myself when I am on stage. This works for me, and I am sure that others have developed their own method for practicing and building their inner confidence when they perform. Nothing wrong with how others do their thing. I am certain most professionals develop a system to be at their best when they have to be.

Review Is Most Important

I have always said that if I do something a hundred times and another person does the same routine ten times, I must be doing it better—all other things being equal, of course. Which means that I and the other person have about the same abilities. We must come up with a program that allows us to do these routines, as a way to review the material we've studied.

Review is one of the keys to getting better. If you review enough, you can learn lyrics to songs. Become a better typist. Be a better baseball player. Stay in good shape. Anything.

Someone once asked me how much time he should spend in review. It's a good question because I'm aware that each of us has a different time schedule. Some people have a day job. Some go to college and must do a great amount of research. Others may have two jobs a day so they can make enough money to support themselves and their family.

Everybody's situation is different and I can't speak specifically here. What I am saying is that we each must find a way to have the time to study and review our craft. I only know how much time I have and how much time I can contribute to my studies, which is at least several hours a day.

I'm certain if each of us searches our time schedules we can come up an idea of how much time we can study and how much time we can practice or review to become what we want to become.

As you investigate your time, you'll learn to prioritize and will discover what works for you. That's how I came up with a concept of what to do with my time and how I can use this time for my development. I'm happy that I did because I have a good block of time for my training, as well as time to spend with my friends and by myself.

I think I have everything in a place in my mind that works for Sam Ulano. You must find what works for you. If you look at yourself hard enough, you will find how to develop your review time on whatever you need to review.

I will say, however, that it is important to spend at least some time in review each and every day. Anything less will not work.

Jot Down Your Ideas, Don't Wait!

I have learned over the years that ideas and interesting thoughts come to all of us. I literally jump out of bed when an idea comes to me! I have a pad of paper nearby and I write these ideas down. I have found over the years that if I wait until later, the idea—no matter how incredible and permanent it seemed at the time—goes away. It disappears. I try to review in my mind what it was I was thinking about, but, for the life of me, I just can't recapture that thought. It always bugs me when this happens.

So for many years now, I write my ideas down that come to me, even if I'm half asleep, because sleep fades my ideas and then I get angry.

In fact, I was sleeping in my bed and awoke to go to the bathroom when the idea for this book came to me. I immediately wrote down about 54 topics that I felt fit into this scheme of things. I wrote the first part of the book in about nine days. Then I gave it to my editor and he did such a wonderful job of making sure that what I wrote was what I meant. He was so helpful and many people have been complimentary to me after reading those first few pages as they "rolled off the press."

About four or five days later, again in my sleep, I got this computer-brain of mine clicking again, and I came up with enough ideas to add the second part of my book. It's just fascinating how the mind works, and I am into writing these pages and topics that I feel fit my Philosophy of Life at 80. I tell everyone that if an idea comes to you, write it down. You may not do anything with it right way, but maybe later on something may click in your brain, and the next thing you know, you may have formulated ideas for a book, lyrics to a song, or an answer to a problem that's been plaguing you.

A friend of mine has a habit of jotting down his dreams. He makes notes and sort of discusses these dreams with himself. Sounds nutty and crazy, but he tells me one of these days he'll sketch his dreams out on his computer. I think that's great, man!

In addition to a pen and pad of paper, have a portable tape machine at your bedside or your work table. You can record your ideas and then have this material transcribed. Now on a computer you can get a print-out and have your ideas right in front of you. But for many years, recording machines were very handy and a secretary would type the letters or whatever it may be on paper, and here once again you have a written record of your thoughts.

So, if there's any tip I can give you at all about making your ideas work, it's to write those thoughts down. Like they say in the Lotto: You never know!

Train Your Memory

I think it is important that you develop your ability to remember people's names, phone numbers, who they are, and what they do. Get to know who you're talking to and where these people fit into your life. In my business I try my best to remember who I'm talking to and as much as I can recall about them whenever our paths cross.

I have friends that can remember many things. If they are in music, they remember songs, the keys the songs are in. They recall the people in the audience that they have met somewhere along the way.

Train your memory to record everything you can about a person. I can remember a person's abilities as a sax man, for instance, or a trumpet player, as well as where we played together, what kind of affair it was and so forth. It's nice to be able to do this. You won't get shot if you don't remember somebody's name, but you might just make a deeper connection with a person if you remember things about them.

I sing about fifty songs and because I am involved with this phase of music, I make it my business to know my keys and other details that are involved in this phase of the music business. I make an effort to remember the names of customers that I meet at the Red Blazer. People appreciate this and are impressed that someone remembers their name, who they are, what kind of work they do, when they were up at the club and just little things. Like the song says: "Little things mean a lot."

As people get older they sometimes lose their memory. This isn't pleasant. Fortunately, I read articles about new research nowadays that say making a conscious effort to remember things—even little things as I discussed earlier—improves your memory and keeps it fresh, no matter how old you get.

I find that at 80 my mind is sharp. I still have control over my brain-computer. And I still work at retaining as many ideas as I can—it doesn't "come naturally." Unfortunately, many people take their memory for granted, and then wonder why it's gone.

Put a Professional-Quality Press Kit Together

A good press kit should tell of your background: where you worked in the past and where you work now. It should highlight any education you've had, in the field of music or otherwise. It should identify your expertise and experience and many other things about your life. Someone reading through a press kit should know if you are in the arts, music, or education and whether you have been recorded.

Also important, you should mention who you studied with and whether you've have written any literature or books in your chosen field. Name the titles and what the books are about. DON'T BE AFRAID TO LIST ALL YOUR ACCOMPLISHMENTS AND WHAT YOU ARE DOING AT THE PRESENT TIME, WHEN YOU'RE AVAILABLE AND WHAT YOUR STRENGTHS ARE.

In planning a press kit, I advise you to include professional photos. However, a big mistake is made by many people when they send out what I call "home photos." Generally, I'm against this practice because rarely do nonprofessional photos show you off to your best.

If you need photos, spend a few bucks and go to a professional photographer and get a series of good quality prints. This is especially important if the photos may be used for an article in a magazine or newspaper. High-quality pictures will have the effect that you look like you are someone who knows what they are doing.

Have your "bio" set on a computer. It should look good, be easy to read, have all the t's crossed and i's dotted, so to speak. Remember, a press kit not only goes out to the media, but to whomever you decide to send it so that it can further your career. As such, a good press kit should be edited by someone who knows how to edit this material.

In preparing your press kit, be prepared to have enough of them so you can send them out and still have copies left for future use. This means you must invest dollars to have this material professionally packaged and ready for the people to whom you are going to send it. This gets back to my saying, "You'll pay the price even if you don't pay the price."

If you have an agent, then include his or her card in the press kit. Possibly, the agent might send out the press kit. He or she may have great connections that can benefit you.

In my 80 years I have learned about this business of music. This doesn't mean I know everything. If you need more advice about putting a press kit together, I suggest you look for someone whose expertise deals with this specialty.

We learn by trial and error. Experiment with how you wish to put your press kit together. Soon, with a little forethought and hard work, you'll be on the road to success.

If You Need Legal Help, Get It

If you are in need of legal help, find a lawyer who knows about the help you need. There are times we need advice and only a person trained in law can help. There have been times when I needed legal help. I found people who were able to help me.

If you do not know where to find this type of help call one of the better law schools and ask them if they can direct you toward the proper legal advice. There are people in all forms of legal advice. I always say that in America we can find what we are looking for. If it is a question of money and you do not have the money to pay for this help, the Legal Aid Society can help you. If you belong to a union, the union should have a legal department that can assist you. As the Bible says, "Seek and thou shall find."

Some instances where it's preferable to use a lawyer's expertise is to make sure a contract is correct. If you need a patent, a lawyer who knows patent law is where you must look for assistance. If you have a band and the band is being signed by a record company, then you need someone who knows this side of the business.

I am not a lawyer and so I don't depend on myself to think I can handle this type of situation. It is best to have someone direct you and to be more certain that you are signing the proper papers and THAT YOU UNDERSTAND WHAT THE LEGAL RAMIFICATIONS ARE.

Don't Be So Quick to Sign on the Dotted Line

I find that I still learn much about the music business. I never thought I knew it all. No one does and BEFORE YOU GET HURT YOU SHOULD GET ADVICE. Contracts especially are very ticklish things, and one must think twice before getting involved and "signing on the bottom line." Even big stars and big companies have problems in these situations, and famous people also must be careful when signing these kinds of documents.

The problem with contracts and other so-called "professional" attachments is that they always appear to be enticing or appealing. Sexy even. When you are young and sort of wet behind the ears, the thought of getting involved with contracts raises all kinds of fantasies. I have learned, however, that it's wise to get professional advice and think twice before signing on the dotted line, no matter how good it sounds at first. I learned this from a very young age. Let me relate a story here..

When I was much younger, my brothers and sisters and mother gave me a great deal of advice. They would tell me how to dress, how to behave, and other general things. Above all, they taught me right from wrong. These are things a young person has to hear and know about. Sort of common sense things. Sound advice.

But when it came to understanding things that involved music, particularly the business end of things, I needed a different kind of advice. One place I found that was the Musician's Union, Local 802 here in New York. (I was a member for 40 years; card number U-78!)

I was out of high school and teaching drums in the Bronx. I had written a great many of my early drum instruction books. I knew enough to copyright my material through the Library of Congress. Mr. Torgman, my drum instructor who was part of the Radio City Music Hall, thought I had written some excellent drum study books. So he set up an appointment for me with one of the big music publishers. I was thrilled and thought this was going to be important to me.

We had a meeting with this publishing company and they had plans to publish my books. There were five particular books involved in this meeting. After awhile they told me that they were going to give me $500 dollars for my five books. In those days, that was considered a lot of money! Then they introduced me to a famous drummer and said that my books would have his name on them, not mine.

I gathered up my written material and told them to go fly a kite and headed back to my drum studio. At that time my eldest brother had a big firm and I decided to call him. He suggested I come down to his place and meet with his company lawyers. I did just that. My brother's legal adviser told me he wasn't a drummer and knew nothing about what I had written. However, he did say to me, "Sam, take this material home, put it in a safe place and in later years you may wish to publish it yourself."

His advice to me was very helpful and I EVENTUALLY PUBLISHED ALL THESE BOOKS UNDER MY OWN NAME.

What I'm saying here is that I learned that legal advice from a good lawyer, which has been very helpful to me. This is why I say, when you need a lawyer's input and someone you can trust, make sure you get it and don't do things without someone who can show you the way.

Here at 80, I have used this advice many times. Not just concerning lawyers, but also doctors, directors and anyone I need that can steer me in the right direction.

The auto industry had a car called Packard and their advertising slogan some years ago was, "Ask the man who owns one and he will tell you." Sometimes slogans like that make sense because there's a lot of truth to them. Talking to someone who knows and using this advice can put you on the right track and save yourself much heartache down the pike.

Learn on the Job

I always thought the best way to learn something was "on the job," hence the term "on-the-job training." My son is in Hollywood and involved with the making of films. Some of his work is for television. He learned his craft while working on the gig.

He must have learned well because he got an Oscar for doing the sound on a small little film you might have heard of—"Titanic." Yes, he's done some of the better movies. He also did "Austin Powers, the Spy That Shagged Me," "Stuart Little," and many other films. At present he does a weekly TV series called "The District." Not too shabby for someone learning his art on the job. He's done well.

So I say get as much information about whatever field you will be involved with. This way you get information and learn what to do and when to do it in this work. I am certain there are people who can direct you and tell you what is needed so you can be professional in your work. Again, as Sy Oliver the bandleader would say, "It's so easy when you know how."

Something I learned how to do long ago was to be on stage. I direct and lead my band. This is my work and how I have made my living. So this is where I can tell people on stage what has to be done. But in other areas of my life, I listen to the director. Simple as that.

In a recording studio making a CD, for instance, I let the sound director tell the band what has to be done. I do not tell the engineer in charge of the recording how to run his studio. I listen like everyone else, in an effort to make the recording sound the best it can be. Like Sinatra said, we all have to take direction and follow orders of the person in charge.

So learn on the job. AND ONE OF THE WAYS TO DO THIS IS TO ASK QUESTIONS OF THOSE AROUND YOU WHO KNOW WHAT IT TAKES. Absorb everything as much as you can. I think they call it "osmosis."

Control Your Anger

Life is too short to lose control of ourselves. Don't get me wrong, I have lost my cool over the years. But, as much as I am able, I catch myself very quickly and ask, "What is so important that I lose control of myself?"

Now, I can't say I always came up with an answer that prevented me from losing a handle on my emotions. No, in fact, there were times I blew my top and felt like I was going to go off the deep end. I didn't like how my body felt in those situations. I gritted my teeth. I felt my blood pressure rise. All in all, I'd allowed some nit-wit get to me.

But the thing I've learned is that, TIME AND AGAIN, WHEN I GAVE IT SOME SERIOUS THOUGHT, I WAS BLOWING STEAM OVER NOTHING. I see it really wasn't over anything so important. I was fired from a band one time after working with the bandleader for seven years. I said things that I look back on now and realize I'd lost control over nonsense.

I will try to never do that again. I strongly believe I'll have better mental control over myself and not allow myself to make such a fool of myself. I would think hard about who I am getting so upset about. I will think better of the language I use. I will ask myself whether this person is so important in my life that he or she is worth having my emotions twisted. And even then, if the answer is yes, I believe it's best not to act in anger. Feel it, but don't act on it. I sit and think about things, then respond accordingly.

As I look back on the times I lost my temper, I know I was just downright stupid. Not wrong to feel that way, maybe, but stupid for letting it adversely affect me the way it did.

Looking back, I feel that, at worst, maybe I'D HAD MY EGO HURT.

Had I taken a step back and seen what I was doing, I probably wouldn't have allowed my blood pressure to rise and explode. Gosh, was I angry! I can see where this anger could lead a person to doing something very dangerous, either to another person or to himself by the way he reacts.

Losing control of our computer-brain, our inner guts, our self-control, can damage our nervous system, heart and other parts of our bodies. I'm not a doctor, but I really believe this. Don't you agree?

Learn from Buddy Rich:
Don't Put Yourself Down

Don't put yourself down. It's not healthy and doesn't accomplish anything for you. In fact it can cut into the confidence of others who like to use your talents. Like my good friend Buddy Rich, the greatest drummer who ever lived (my opinion), once said to me, we must like ourselves first before we get others to like us. I agree with him all the way.

Buddy Rich passed away about 13 years ago, and I considered him a dear friend of mine. He was an inspiring force. He was confident and probably the greatest talent on a set of drums.

Others for years thought he was conceited and arrogant and all the other nonsense. No way. He was sure and definite and was always in control when it came to his drumming skills. There never was anybody like him. I doubt if there ever will be someone like Buddy Rich. I never heard him put himself down. I always heard him be sure. This quality showed on his face.

Many didn't like him, but that's their problem. Maybe they were jealous of his great skills and abilities. I don't know, but I saw only the virtuosity of this man. He was the master of his abilities. Never did I see him falter. Never did I see him not play well. His worst was everyone else's best. He was that good.

IF I EVER LEARNED ANYTHING FROM BUDDY RICH, IT WAS NOT TO TEAR YOURSELF DOWN. NO FALSE MODESTY. Like what you do, think about what you do, try to always be your very best. He personified this attitude. He had complete control and confidence in his talents and abilities.

For those who didn't meet or know Buddy Rich, he played with Artie Shaw's band in 1937. I found it interesting when I asked Buddy, about two years before he died, whether he could play all the great Artie Shaw big band arrangements now as he did in years gone by. Without hesitation he said, "Sam, I could play them better now!"

At my age of 80, I never am unhappy with my nightly performance. I've learned that what I do is what I do at that time and so I accept it. That's all. Criticizing myself after I've done what I've done isn't going to help me.

Putting yourself down is not the style of a true professional, and we must avoid doing this in our life. Being sure in what you do is most important. I am more certain than ever about what I can do in my band and in my educational work. I think many of us should learn that putting ourselves down is not good for us.

Never Quit

This has always been one of my main mottos. I tell myself anyone can quit, but not everyone can complete what they start out to do. How many of us have started a diet and never followed it through to where we lost the weight we wanted? I know it isn't easy; there are many obstacles in our way. That's why it's easier to quit than to persevere. Quitting is the easy way out.

There have been times in my life that I thought about quitting. But I continued straight ahead and kept plugging at what I was doing. Like writing a new drum instruction book. Finishing a recording project. Making reprints of older publications so I keep them in print. Whatever it was I was doing, I said to myself, "I'm never going to quit."

I have students who started writing a new study book and almost finish it. I'll say, "What happened to your book?" And they'll say, "I had things I had to do and the book is on the back burner." A year or two later, I'll ask again. And they'll answer, "My mother got sick." Or they'll say, "I had to go on the road...I was sick...My day gig got very busy." On and on it went.

I could write a book of all the reasons, excuses, all of the road-blocks that got in everyone's way. It's very common. HOW MANY OF US DROPPED OUT OF COLLEGE? HOW MANY JUST COULDN'T SEE THE END OF THE TUNNEL? HOW MANY PEOPLE STARTED TO DO SOMETHING THAT WAS IMPORTANT TO THEM, THAT THEY WOULD HAVE LOVED TO FINISH AND NEVER DID?

I never understood this. I try to finish everything I start, even if I am the only one who will like what I did. I make it my business to complete what I start, and that is what makes me happy about my life. I have asked a few people if they have any plans to finish things they started and how are they coming along with what they are doing. They come up with some crazy excuses. Too bad.

The fun of writing my Philosophy of Life at 80 is that I enjoy doing this project, and I am getting satisfaction and happiness from the book.

What else is there in life except the enjoyment of doing nice things? This project doesn't cost me big bucks and every day I add another piece to the puzzle.

Never quit. Never say to yourself that you're tired of whatever it is you're doing. Finish it. Put it aside if you must, but then come back and look at what you did. As for me, this book of mine has given me great pleasure. But it will be even more rewarding once it's done. Because I didn't quit.

It's Never Too Late

Someone once asked me if it was ever too late in life to start studying the piano or take up the drums. It's a very common question: "When is it too late?" I always give the same answer: "Never!" It is never too late, and as soon as people realize this, they may find enjoyment in their lives.

If you read some of the senior citizen magazines, you'll find out how many elderly people have discovered it is never too late to do something with their lives. Learn to play golf. Travel all around the world. Relocate to Florida, Arizona, California or wherever their dreams will take them. No, it is never too late.

A nice lady friend makes the most gorgeous quilts. Just marvelous. She also sings quite nicely. She just turned 71, and here's the kicker, SHE HAS A SIX-DAYS-A-WEEK JOB AS A WAITRESS!

I'm 80 and have been practicing my drums, playing a couple nights a week and still teaching a few students every week. I have found a great deal to do with my life. Sometimes I am amazed how so many of us are just living to die.

It is never too late. My sister is 83. A few years ago, she went back to college and took a jazz course, out in California.

It's never too late. Grandma Moses was up there in age when she started to paint. Others have climbed mountains, gone sky diving, taken dancing lessons. Many people find new hobbies at all ages. Yes, there is so much to do and all one has to do is get inspired and start to develop these new ideas in life.

No, I say, it's never too late in life to find something to do.

It's not even too late to start lifting weights. (But, hey, like I've said a dozen times already, see your doctor before starting any physical exercise already!) You don't need to do lot of weight. A steady, daily program, 20 to 30 minutes a day.

No people, it is never too late. Give yourself a chance to investigate this concept. Tell yourself, "It is never too late!"

As You Get Older, You Get Better

I have noticed that as we get older, we get better in our craft. And because we get better, we know more and can be important to our profession. This makes our value much greater.

We see it in all fields of endeavor. Most of the time we look for people with experience in what they do, be it government, the military, or big business. People who have knowledge and are trained become the head honchos in most fields.

I found that as I got older and more experienced as a drummer and educator, more and more people would seek me out to study with me. Of course this doesn't mean that this will happen all the time, but I see it more and more each day. I'm often called by excellent players who need more instruction and more direction in order to become better drummers.

Notice that the youngsters are not the principals in schools and colleges. Coaches of sports teams are older than the players on the team.

So I say that as we get older, we are the people that younger people seek to learn from. As I reflect on my life, I realize I really knew very little about my instrument in my younger days. As I matured, practiced, studied and advanced as a player, writer, educator and lecturer, I developed my skills. So here I am looking back on my career, and I know more than ever that as we age, we get better.

Recognize Your Faults
So You Can Correct Them

Eventually, we come to recognize our faults. Once we know this about ourselves, we then can try to correct them.

Years ago I used to smoke and never realized how bad my breath was, or how I was a sloppy smoker. I'd get ashes on my clothes, on the floor, and even would mess up other people's homes. Eventually I knew I didn't want to smoke, for this and many other reasons. On top of everything, it was costing me hard-earned money.

A little less than 40 years ago, I stopped smoking cigarettes cold turkey and have never smoked since.

However, I started to smoke cigars. It was fashionable and I thought I liked the cigar. But this too became something that I didn't enjoy and I gave it up as well. I didn't like the bad odor in my mouth, and I wouldn't like the way my food tasted. One time, I burned a hole in an expensive cashmere coat. That was it. Out went the cigars and nowadays I can't stand the smell of cigars or cigarettes. I never went back to smoking.

I don't like the smell of liquor either, and I know that drinking wasn't for me. As I wrote earlier, I never have been drunk and never liked social drinking or having one at one of my gigs. I think if I drank all the booze that has been offered to me at the many clubs I work, I'd be a hopeless alcoholic. That's not for me, and I have stayed away from drinking all my musical life. This goes back to before I was in the army.

I am certain I have many other faults. But, little by little, I HAVE MADE AN EFFORT TO CORRECT THEM AND MAKE SURE I DON'T FALL VICTIM TO THESE FAULTS AGAIN.

I always suggest to my drum students that they make an honest list of their faults. Such as not paying their bills. Their rent. Answering their mail. Putting off things they must do and procrastinating, and whatever else they consider their faults to be.

Remind yourself of your faults and make every effort to work them out. You might find that you are happier for it. I always say it can be done. We just need to make the effort to work them out of our life.

Try Never to Make the Same Mistake

We all make mistakes. In fact we may make the same mistake many times. We try not to make the same goofs too often, but it's only human nature: We do things, we make mistakes. Eventually we find ways not to make these errors.

I look at things a little differently. I don't call mistakes "mistakes."

To me there is a way to do something and there is a way not to do it. I don't call them errors or mistakes; I just say they are things that don't match what needs to be done to get the job done. If what we do doesn't work, we must try to do certain things a different way.

I try to study what I did and go over the things I consider not the best method to do what I did. Eventually I find the proper way to do things. If you are not happy with a "mistake," study what it is that you don't like. You will find the correct way that you seek.

Many of us are bothered by mistakes. Many of us criticize ourselves. This can be very upsetting. We shouldn't allow ourselves to be affected by mistakes. If we allow these mistakes to get into our system, before you know it we start to make these errors even more. It throws us out of whack and it really sets us up for serious troubles.

Just see mistakes for what they are, and ask yourself: is this way of doing something working? If not, consider it an excellent opportunity to learn a new approach to a problem.

Persevere!

If you don't stick with things, then no results can show up. If you plug away every day, little by little, you'll see something form. This will give you something to work with, and hopefully you'll see it through to the finish.

Many times you may not like the finished results. Sometimes you may be discouraged by the results. No problem. We don't have to like everything we do. However, in maybe a year or so we may look back at what we did, and our mind may just find ways to change what we did. And this change may be just what we need to make the finished work better.

I look back to when I was 15 years old and wrote some of my first drum instruction material. At that age, I had no idea how good the material I sketched out was. As I got older and better in my craft as a drummer, I started looking back at my early writings and there I saw the beginning of my first instruction book. IT BECAME KNOWN AS "BASS BOPS" AND HERE IN THE YEAR OF 2001, THIS BOOK HAS STOOD THE TEST OF TIME. The book has always been in print and drummers all over have studied from my first book. I actually wrote it in 1935—when I was 15—and first published it in 1948. I was, and still am, proud of that first book.

My family thought I was nuts and over the years had no idea that I had this kind of talent to play drums and teach and write and perform. Like all families, many never know when someone in their family has the ability to be a professional.

My motto is, "Stick with it. Results will come." I really do believe this. I feel that if I give it my best shot and stick with what I love to do; continue to practice and study; and, above all, never let these things go, then results will show up. They have shown up and they will continue to show up.

This sounds like I am a fanatic, and maybe I am—I think we have to be fanatical and stick with what we want and love to do. I say that this is the real test of one's abilities.

Start something and stick with it. All the heartaches, all the disappointments, all the difficulties that go with trying to develop our talents and trying to be somebody—all this pays off as time goes by.

You have to believe in yourself, and if you believe, then give it a real try by sticking with it.

Don't Feel Sorry for Yourself

I think one of the worst things you can do is to feel sorry for yourself. No one else will feel sorry for you, and feeling this way is not an answer to solve how you feel.

I'm certain that we all have times when we are down in the dumps and it takes a little while for this feeling goes away. I know it's a normal reaction to things that happen to us. But this down feeling sometimes can be very dangerous.

Some of us might be depressed at times like this. I have experienced this feeling of self-pity, and I don't have a secret cure to this feeling sorry for myself. I wish I did have an answer. I usually tell myself this low and miserable feeling will eventually go away. In my experience, it can linger for some days, but I have noticed that it disappears and I feel great again.

I guess what I'm saying is that I accept this emotion and allow it to ride itself out of my system. I really must say that I don't have this sorry feeling very often anymore. I think it's part of human nature. Go with the flow. I AM CERTAIN THAT THIS FEELING SORRY FOR ONESELF GOES ALONG WITH LIVING LIFE.

What brings this on? Who knows. As I said I very seldom feel this way and my best cure is to ride it out. I'll brood about it for a day or less and let myself try to understand just what caused me to have this down feeling. Did I do something, or am I avoiding another feeling that brought it on? I like to study myself and what makes me tick.

I have found that sometimes I had high expectations, and these high thoughts didn't work out, and the next thing

I knew I was feeling sorry for myself. Feeling this way did-n't help me, and as I began to understand myself, I knew I had to find a better answer. Basically, I stopped feeling sorry for myself. While this in itself didn't make me feel better, it at least didn't compound the problem, and I was able to focus on other things.

See What You Did in the Past

What you did in the past can be very valuable to you as you grow older. I look back on my writing and performances I took part in and even write down a sort of diary of what I did and what's happening in my life. Sometimes these flashbacks help me write a new book or improve my talent.

Many people base their memoirs on what they did in their lives. You can tell when you read through this book, for example, that it's what my life has been about and how I came to my conclusions of what life in general is about.

If you review your past and what you did in your years, you too might come up with an interesting book about your life. This can be your ideas about life. How you see life and what makes you happy about what you did in years gone by.

I started to think about my life and what I've accomplished during the years. I realized what the main reasons were that I was able to do these things: I stayed in good physical shape, I incorporated a system, and so forth.

This has been fun for me because I can look back and study what I have done and what else I wish to do with my life. I am not yet ready to retire, and so studying what I did and still can do is very valuable to me.

My mind is still fertile and still thinks of what there is to write about and what new adventures I am capable of exploring. This makes me happy and it also keeps my brain alive and active.

I understand life a lot better now, and I still have the direction I wish to go in. You would be surprised at how many of my friends are undecided about what to do with their lives, and they just keep growing older. Somehow they have lost their purpose for living and enjoying their lives.

So observing my past gives me some idea as to how I can continue with my life and be productive.

Don't 'Fluff' Anyone Off

In my 80 years of life, I have learned one of the great things is to never ignore anyone, to never "fluff anyone off" as they used to say.

Many times, especially in sports or music, I'll read that some guy or gal wouldn't sign autographs or wouldn't say hello to their fans or peers. That behavior is not good for your reputation. We don't need others to pass the word around that this baseball player, or actor, or whatever field a performer is in, fluffs their fans off. This can come back to haunt you. I always say it is tough enough to build a good name, so who needs to be known in the negative!

I have never heard anyone say nasty things about Gene Krupa. Or Louie Bellson. Only nice things were said about these two particular drummers. I have been outspoken in my field for many years; however, I have never ignored students, new talents and people that like to pick my brain. I listen and I try to be fair and give the person talking to me all my attention.

I know many people in all fields that have reputations of being someone who doesn't like to answer questions or say things that shouldn't be said. However, I do speak my mind. I feel that if it's true, I am not afraid to say it. I know many times when I am involved in conversations, I speak my mind to most musicians or the owner of a club I am working. I don't hold back. I find that I would be very unhappy if I held back and didn't say what I had to say.

Ignoring people, refusing to give an autograph, not being a good listener even when you think this is not the time to be a good listener—YOU HAVE TO APPRAISE THE SIT-

UATION AND JUDGE FOR YOURSELF IF IT COMES UNDER THE HEADING OF FLUFFING SOMEONE OFF. But if you do feel like you've fluffed someone off, it's never too late to make amends. There are times you can apologize after the incident or, if you know the person, pick up the phone and call that person. Do it gracefully—the way you would have liked to have handled the situation in the first place.

Do What You Can Do,
Not What You Can't

Someone once said that as we grow older, we should continue to learn about ourselves. I agree with this. One of the most important things I have learned about myself is to never try to do things I'm not capable of doing. I stick within my abilities. This means I try to know how far my talents can take me.

As long as I really know to what extent I can go, I never get hurt. For example, I've written quite a few drum instruction books and I've published them myself. However, I don't try to have the book printed when I'm not certain of the material. Just to have another book out is not the goal.

The material must add something to the study of drums. It must have a purpose and it must be clear and well explained. This way, I feel my literature will be understood by people far away. This way, the book will make sense to me, and the students, teachers and professionals will understand what I am writing about.

The next thing I must have is the dollars to publish this new work. I don't want to be in debt and owe the printer, or an editor or whatever other costs may be involved. I hate owing money, and so when I have the cash or the money in my bank, I do what I can.

Years ago, I overspent and found myself always owing money. I don't want that to happen, and I don't want stretch my pocketbook so that later on I'll have trouble. Once I learned this control, I was happy and all set to do the things I wanted to do. Many of my friends will go into debt and suffer for it.

Even in my playing, I don't try to reach for things that are not in my musical abilities. I study myself and know just how well I can do what is in my grasp. This too makes me happy, and I know how to play at the level that makes sense to me.

In my business of music this problem is called "overplaying." So I try to stay within my talents. It works for me. So if you haven't learned this yet, I say you better understand yourself and know how far you can go.

As Kenny Rogers sang, "Know When to Hold 'Em; Know When to Fold 'Em"

This is such a great statement. In other words, quit while you're ahead—or even when you're behind, for that matter! Friends of mine go to Atlantic City, win some money, then stick around long enough to lose it again—plus some of their own money! Not such a good idea.

These people are not real gamblers, mostly because they never learned to stop when they are ahead. It's not easy to learn this control, but if you don't wish to get hurt, you have to learn that there is a time to stick around and a time to pack it in. I have that ability to say to myself, "Sam, go home—now!"

What a great feeling it is to be able to talk to myself and say enough is enough. When I get home I say that I can always go back another day. I'm not a habitual gambler, but I like the feeling of winning some money and being able to stop, dead cold, at that time.

When I gave up smoking cigarettes many years ago, I stopped cold turkey. The same for smoking cigars. I had the willpower to never drink and never experienced what it was like to be drunk. I saw too many people drink and become basket cases.

I was able to resist drugs. Never experimented to see what it was like. I didn't allow peer pressure to convince me that I had to try something because I was afraid of what my friends would say if I didn't.

I listened to Kenny Rogers' lyrics: "You gotta know when to hold 'em; know when to fold 'em. Know when to walk away; know when to run."

I never wanted to push myself to the edge. Fortunately, I learned this as a young person, and now I never regret that I didn't try various dangerous things in my life. At 80, my body feels great, my mind is clear, and I think I'll make it to 90. Who knows, 100 doesn't seem too far-fetched!

Never Spend Money You Don't Have

In my younger days, I owned a drum shop in the Bronx. I sold drums, drum parts and also taught lessons to aspiring young artists. This goes back quite a few years. I had a great stock of drum supplies and was doing well.

Many of my customers would owe me some bucks. In fact, it became quite a few dollars owed to me. These customers would call me up and say they are sending out a check to pay for the supplies they purchased from me. So I was expecting some good amount of change to be in my mailbox the next day or so. I would jump the gun and send out a check to pay for material I needed in my store. However, I didn't have that money in the bank to cover the checks I sent out. I was anticipating money to come in.

Guess what happened? I didn't get the money promised to me and in the meantime, the people I'd written checks to deposited them and—boom!—my checks bounced. I then made all kinds of excuses: "The bank made a mistake!...Somebody else's check must have bounced!...I made an error in my bookkeeping!"...and on and on.

Bullshit! I'd spent money I didn't have.

I LEARNED THAT LESSON THE HARD WAY AND SOON I BECAME A BETTER BUSINESS PERSON BECAUSE I NEVER HAD THAT HAPPEN TO ME AGAIN. No more liberal credit policies and no more bounced checks!

You can't spend what you don't have, nor what you're expecting to have. Unless you're ready for trouble.

Don't Overexercise

I wrote earlier on the importance of keeping your body in top shape. I try to get people to understand the value of why you should keep yourself in the best of condition.

Now here's the flip side of the coin: If you *overexercise*, you will get burned out. Some people call it "overtraining."

If you go to a gym, you are taught to work out a day, skip a day, work out a day, skip a day, and so on. Some gyms have people work out three days a week, skipping every other day. Some gyms have people work out almost every day, but they work on different body parts—never the same part of the body two days in a row.

There are many variations on how to train the body. If people want to bulk up, get big biceps or more defined stomach muscles, you eat and train a certain way.

I spent 13 years at Sigmond Klien's gym. Interestingly, he told most of us not to go to a gym. He told us to buy our own free weights and follow his program at our homes. That was the best advice! I have stuck with Sigmond's program.

Another thing Sigmond taught me was the value of not overtraining. Overdoing your training will burn out your muscles, and this can be dangerous and do damage.

So I tell everyone it is important to have someone teach them how to train with weights and how to develop a body condition system that keeps you strong. Sigmond's advice was short practice routines: Do each exercise for ten repetitions. If you are just starting out, stick with these ten reps for three to six months. Allow your body to develop control and feel the strength you develop in your arms, legs, back, midriff. As I wrote earlier, I use 10-,15- and 20-pound free weights. This has worked for me.

Keep it simple, control your desire to do more, and you'll find more is not better. Take it from me. Moderation. Simplicity.

There Is Always Someone to Learn From

Every day I meet someone who tells me they are always learning something new. I feel the same way. There is always someone who has ideas that I can pick up.

I talk to people who are always telling me that they have picked up some ideas that have helped them. I have run across drummers in my field who have ideas I never heard or saw that I was able to use in my work. It's interesting because this is an ongoing thing. New inventions for my instrument!

A new book just came out that showed me another way to do something I never did. It's incredible how this works.

I started to realize as I got older that I had to always study. I practice as much now on my instrument and feel I am studying even harder than when I was 50 or younger. I'm glad that I do this because it keeps me sharp and on top of my abilities. I made a vow to myself to always stay in tip-top shape. I think it's easy to do. All we have to do is put our minds to it.

In my field I try to go to as many clinics or seminars as my schedule allows. Even though I may hear things that I know about and have heard others talk about, this rehashing of ideas is good for me. It also makes me aware that I can't take things for granted.

I would be very unhappy if I allowed myself to get stale and let my drumming skills slide. I've worked too hard all these years to improve these skills. It would make me feel terrible, and I don't like that feeling and will not give in to neglecting my talent.

I talk to people in my field. I listen to others about how they keep their skills up. I ask questions of everyone, even though they may not play the same instrument I do. Hell, they might not even be musicians. I want to know how they develop new ideas in their line of work.

Sometimes it isn't formal study, like going to school or seeing a private teacher. I get satisfaction from hearing others explain what their day gig is like. How they got started in their job and how they study.

Never doubt that you can learn from anybody—even if you learn what not to do!

Like the Song Says,
Put on a Happy Face

I know this sounds easy to do, but enjoying your life brings happiness. And that's a great feeling. Other people pick up on when we are happy and feel better too. My mother had a great philosophy about life. She said, "Every day we live, we should enjoy it."

That to me is such a marvelous statement. Think about that. My mom also said that facing each day, with its challenges and working them out, is the fun of living.

Makes sense to me. I know each day can be difficult to live through if things are not going our way. But nothing is too important to brood about, to be down on ourselves. I always say, "Give tomorrow a shot; it may be a great day!" Nothing is so terrible that we should get so depressed that we can't face the next day.

I read once where a very famous person was asked the first thing he did when he woke up in the morning. As I remember his quote, it went something like this: "The first thing I do is to read the obituary column, and if I don't see my name, I get up and have a wonderful day."

All of this sounds so simple as I type it out. We must find what we love to do with our lives. We then must proceed to try and accomplish what we want to do with ourselves. I see this as fun.

If we live within our means; if we don't try to do things that we are not ready to do and keep progressing in our talents then, man, this is such a wonderful world to live in!

As Louie Armstrong, the great jazz musician sang on one of his hit records, "What a Wonderful World." To me that song says it all, with such a great melody and wonderful lyrics. It's also one of the most requested songs we get every night we perform.

If you think about this, we come through this life one time and then we are gone for a long while. So the time we spend in this world, we should have a grand time. Make life a blast and be happy inside yourself.

Put on that happy face. The song says when you're smiling, the whole world smiles with you; when you're laughing, the whole world laughs with you. What a wonderful world!

Sam Ulano is often described as having the ability to "open your mind and make you think." Whether through his music or his witticisms about life, Sam brings a unique approach to living. Taking up the drums at age 13, Sam opened his first studio four years later and began teaching and writing about the drums. He followed up high school with four years at the Manhattan School of Music before being drafted into the army, where he trained a 100-piece drum corps.

Now 80 years old and showing no signs of letting up, Sam is a performer, educator and author who has been in the music profession for over 65 years. During that time, he has studied with and taught the best of them, while carving out a niche for himself as a respected drummer on the New York scene. Sam has played at many of the top nightspots in New York, including the Gaslight Club and, currently, the famed Red Blazer. He's played the summer resorts, the concert field, and is known as "Mr. Rhythm" for his more than 500 shows for young audiences throughout the New York school system. He has appeared on television with Steve Allen on *The Tonight Show*, as well as with Gary Moore, Ernie Kovacs, and Joe Franklin.

Well-known for his methods of drum teaching and his progressive approach to writing about the instrument he loves, Sam has over 2500 instruction books to his credit—300 in the past five years alone! He also has produced records, audio and video tapes, and CDs of his instruction and performance. He continues to write, teach, and perform in his own inimitable style.

Manuscript editor **Ed Petoniak** is a writer and editor living in New York. Born and raised in suburban New Jersey, Ed grew up a Mets fan. Fortunately, this allegiance did not cost him the opportunity to work with Sam, a lifelong Yankees fan. "Sam's chapter on how to handle defeat really came in useful after the World Series," Ed says. "In fact, I'm hoping that Sam gets to use it next year!"

Ed has written about sports, medicine and music. His editing work includes books on neurology, Shakespeare, and the African-American athlete.